# CONTENTS

# IMMUNE BOOSTING SMOOTHIES

## Ultimate Cold And Flu Fighting Smoothie

Servings: 1
Cooking Time: 5 Minutes
**Ingredients:**
- 1 large banana, fresh or frozen
- 2 oranges, peeled and chopped
- 2 cups baby spinach
- Freshly squeezed juice of ½ lemon
- 2 tablespoon Chia seeds (soaked)
- 1 teaspoon of freshly grated ginger
- ¼ cup of filtered water

**Directions:**
1. Whizz all the ingredients in the blender until smooth and serve.

**Nutrition Info:** (Per Serving): Calories- 330, Fat- 5.8 g, Protein-8 g, Carbohydrates-72 g

## Mixed Fruit Magic Smoothie

Servings: 2
Cooking Time: 2 Minutes
**Ingredients:**
- 1 up mixed berries (fresh or frozen)
- 1 banana, chopped (frozen)
- ½ cup fresh pineapple juice
- ½ cup fresh orange juice
- ½ cup low fat yogurt, plain

**Directions:**
1. Place all the ingredients listed above in the same order, one by one into your blender and whip it up on high speed until thick and creamy consistency is got.

**Nutrition Info:** (Per Serving): Calories-140, Fat-2.5 g, Proteins-3.5 g, Carbohydrates- 30 g

## Strawberry-ginger Tea Smoothie

Servings: 1
Cooking Time: 5 Minutes
**Ingredients:**
- 1 cup freshly brewed ginger tea (warm or hot)
- ½ cup strawberries, tops removed
- 1 oranges, peeled and chopped
- ½ line, peeled and chopped
- Juice of ½ lemon
- ¼ teaspoon of freshly grated ginger
- 1 clove of garlic
- A pinch of cayenne pepper
- ¼ teaspoon of cinnamon powder
- 1 teaspoon coconut oil
- 2 tablespoons raw, organic honey
- A pinch of sea salt
- 4-5 cubes of ice (optional)

**Directions:**
1. Prepare a cup of ginger tea and keep it aside.
2. Add all the ingredients into your blender except the tea and process it for a minute.
3. Then add the tea and pulse it for another minute or until well blended.

**Nutrition Info:** (Per Serving): Calories- 210, fat- 5 g, Protein- 1 g, Carbohydrates- 50 g

## Coco-maca Smoothie

Servings: 1
Cooking Time: 5 Minutes
**Ingredients:**
- 1 cup coconut milk,
- 1 banana (fresh or frozen)
- A handful of mixed berries
- 1 teaspoon coconut oil
- ½ teaspoon vanilla extract
- ½ tablespoon Cacao powder
- 1 tablespoon Chia seeds
- ½ teaspoon raw, organic honey or liquid stevia (optional)

**Directions:**
1. Load your blender with all the ingredients and pulse it up until there are no more lumps.

**Nutrition Info:** (Per Serving): Calories-285, Fat-7 g, Protein-21 g, Carbohydrates-40 g

## Cacao- Spirulina And Berry Booster

Servings: 1
Cooking Time: 5 Minutes
**Ingredients:**
- 1 banana, (fresh or frozen)
- 1 cup coconut milk
- 1 cup strawberries (fresh or frozen)
- 1 cup mixed greens
- ½ cup blueberries (frozen)
- 1 teaspoon cacao powder
- 1 teaspoon Spirulina powder
- ½ tablespoon coconut oil
- A large pinch of cinnamon powder
- 1 teaspoon of raw, organic honey,
- 1 tablespoon of any super food of your choice 9 mace, goji berry, bee pollen, aloe, hemp etc.)

**Directions:**
1. Load your smoothie blender with all the mentioned ingredients and pulse it on high speed for 2 minutes.
2. Pour into a glass and enjoy.

**Nutrition Info:** (Per Serving): Calories- 390, Fat- 18 g , Protein- 15 g, Carbohydrates- 50 g

## Papaya Passion

Servings: 1
Cooking Time: 2 Minutes
**Ingredients:**
- 1 cup papaya, chopped
- ½ cup pineapple, peeled and chopped
- 1 cup, low fat or fat free yogurt (plain)
- 1 teaspoon coconut oil
- 1 teaspoon flaxseed powder
- A handful of ice

**Directions:**
1. Add the papaya, pineapple and ice into your blender and process it on medium high speed till well combined.

2. Next add the coconut oil, flaxseed powder and yogurt and process it on high speed for 1 minutes till you get a creamy, thick mixture.
3. Serve chilled!
**Nutrition Info:** (Per Serving): Calories-300, Fat-1.5 g, Protein- 13 g, Carbohydrates- 65 g

## Kiwi- Banana Healer

Servings: 1
Cooking Time: 5 Minutes
**Ingredients:**
- 1 kiwi, peeled and chopped
- ¼ avocado, chopped
- 1 Swiss chard leaf,
- 1 small frozen banana
- 1 cup coconut water
- 1 teaspoon Spirulina powder
- 2 tablespoon hemp seeds
- 3-4 ice cubes

**Directions:**
1. Add all the ingredients one by one into your blender and process until smooth.
**Nutrition Info:** (Per Serving): Calories- 365, Fat-14 g, Protein- 11 g, carbohydrates- 47 g

## Popoye's Pear Smoothie For Kids

Servings: 1
Cooking Time: 5 Minutes
**Ingredients:**
- 1 pear, diced
- ½ avocado
- 1 kiwi, peeled and chopped
- A handful of baby spinach
- A few mixed berries

**Directions:**
1. Wash all the produce thoroughly and add them to the blender.
2. Process it for 1 minute or until well combined.
3. Serve.
**Nutrition Info:** (Per Serving): Calories-320, Fat-15 g, Protein-4 g, Carbohydrates-50 g

## Blueberry Peach Smoothie

Servings: 1
Cooking Time: 5 Minutes
**Ingredients:**
- 1 cup almond milk
- 1 cup peach, cubed (fresh or frozen)
- A handful of blueberries (fresh or frozen)
- 1 cup greens of your choice (kale, spinach)
- 1 tablespoon of Chia seeds
- ½ teaspoon of freshly grated ginger
- 1 tablespoon of any super food of your choice
- 1 tablespoon coconut oil

**Directions:**
1. Add all the ingredients to the blender jar except the coconut oil and process for 1 minute.

2.   Then pour in the oil and blend again for 30 seconds and serve.
**Nutrition Info:** (Per Serving): Calories- 280, Fat- 18 g, Protein- 3 g, Carbohydrates- 34 g

## Yogi-berry Smoothie

Servings: 1
Cooking Time: 5 Minutes
**Ingredients:**
- 2 cups mixed greens of your choice
- 1 cup pineapple, chopped
- ½ orange, peeled and chopped
- 1 kiwi, peeled and chopped
- ½ cup mixed berries (fresh or frozen)
- ½ cup low fat Greek yogurt (plain)
- 1 tablespoon flax seeds (soaked or ground)
- ½ cup filtered water

**Directions:**
1.   To your blender, add all the smoothie ingredients listed above and process until smooth and creamy.
**Nutrition Info:** (Per Serving): Calories-330, Fat-3.4 g, Protein-18.4 g, Carbohydrates- 162 g

## Pomegranate- Berry Smoothie

Servings: 1
Cooking Time: 2 Minutes
**Ingredients:**
- ¾ cup freshly squeezed pomegranate juice
- 1 cups mixed berries (fresh or frozen)
- 1 cup low fat yogurt
- 2-3 drops of vanilla extract
- 1 teaspoon Chia seeds

**Directions:**
1.   Add all the above ingredients into your blender jar and pulse until thick and frothy.
**Nutrition Info:** (Per Serving): Calories- 283, Fat-3 g, Protein-7 g, Carbohydrates-58 g

## Citrus Spinach Immune Booster

Servings: 2
Cooking Time: 5 Minutes
**Ingredients:**
- 1 orange, peeled, deseeded and chopped
- 1 lime, peeled, deseeded and chopped
- A small handful of spinach leaves, washed
- 1-2 peaches, peeled and chopped
- 2 carrots, peeled and chopped
- 1 ½ cups almond milk (unsweetened)

**Directions:**
1.   Dump all the ingredients into the blender and whip it up until the smoothie is thick and creamy.
**Nutrition Info:** (Per Serving): Calories-145, Fat-2g, Protein- 4 g, Carbohydrates- 30 g

## Berry Carrot Smoothie

Servings: 1

Cooking Time: 2 Minutes

**Ingredients:**

- ¾ cup of freshly squeezed orange juice
- ½ cup of low fat plain yogurt
- 1 small carrot, chopped
- 1 cup mixed berries (preferably frozen)
- 2 tablespoon pumpkin seeds

**Directions:**

1. Just add all the ingredients into your blender jar and process the smoothie until it's nice and frothy.

**Nutrition Info:** (Per Serving): Calories- 159, Fat- 5 g, Protein- 4 g, Carbohydrates- 25 g

## Berrilicious Chiller

Servings: 2

Cooking Time: 5 Minutes

**Ingredients:**

- 1 ½ cup mixed berries (fresh or frozen)
- 1 tablespoon freshly squeezed lemon juice
- 6 ounces of unsweetened almond milk
- 2 teaspoons of freshly grated ginger
- 1 tablespoon flax seeds
- 1 ½ tablespoons of raw organic honey
- A handful of ice cubes

**Directions:**

1. Add all the ingredients into your blender and process until smooth and frothy.
2. Serve and enjoy immediately.

**Nutrition Info:** (Per Serving): Calories- 110, Fat-1.5 g, Protein- 1 g, Carbs-26 g

## Orange Coco Smoothie

Servings: 2

Cooking Time: 10 Minutes

**Ingredients:**

- 1 cup freshly squeezed orange juice
- 6 California tangerines, peeled and chopped
- 1 cup mixed greens
- 2 teaspoons freshly grated ginger root
- Juice of 2 freshly squeezed lemons
- 1 ½ cups of coconut milk/ coconut water (your choice)
- 4 teaspoons pure coconut oil
- 2 tablespoons Chia seeds
- 4 teaspoons raw organic honey
- 1 tablespoons any super food of your choice

**Directions:**

1. To your blender jar, add all the ingredients in the given order and whirr it up for 90 seconds or until done.

**Nutrition Info:** (Per Serving): Calories-267, Fat-1.3 g, Protein-5.3 g, Carbohydrates- 68.4 g

## Flaxseed And Berry Smoothie

Servings: 1

Cooking Time: 2 Minutes

**Ingredients:**

- 1 apple, cored and chopped
- ½ cup blueberries (fresh or frozen)
- 2 tablespoons of flaxseeds
- 1/ teaspoon of cinnamon powder
- 1/2 teaspoon of freshly squeezed lemon juice
- ¼ cup of plain fat free yogurt
- 1 teaspoon of raw organic honey
- 1 cup filtered water

**Directions:**

1. Place all the above ingredients into the blender jar and process until the mixture is thick and creamy.

**Nutrition Info:** (Per Serving): Calories- 210, Fat- 6 g, Protein- 5 g, Carbohydrates- 40 g

# DETOX AND CLEANSE SMOOTHIES

## Minty Mango Delight

Servings: 2
Cooking Time: 5 Minutes
**Ingredients:**
- 1 cup freshly squeezed carrot juice
- 2 cups mango, peeled and chopped
- 1 cup freshly squeezed orange juice
- ¼ cup fresh mint, washed
- A pinch of cayenne pepper
- A few ice cubes

**Directions:**
1. Add all the ingredients to your blender jar and process until thick and creamy.

**Nutrition Info:** (Per Serving): Calories- 225, Fat- 0 g, Protein- 3 g, Carbohydrates- 55 g

## Chamomile Ginger Detox Smoothie

Servings: 2
Cooking Time: 10 Minutes
**Ingredients:**
- 3 tablespoons collard greens
- 1 tablespoon chamomile flowers, dried
- 1 pear, chopped
- 1 cantaloupe, sliced and chopped
- ½ inch ginger, peeled
- ½ lemon, juiced
- 1 cup ice
- 1 cup of water

**Directions:**
1. Add all the listed ingredients to a blender
2. Blend until smooth
3. Serve chilled and enjoy!

**Nutrition Info:** Calories: 86; Fat: 0g; Carbohydrates: 22g; Protein: 2g

## Strawberry And Watermelon Medley

Servings: 2
Cooking Time: 5 Minutes
**Ingredients:**
- 1 cup ice
- 1 tablespoon fresh basil
- 1 cup watermelon, cubed
- 1 cup frozen strawberries, cubed
- 1 cup unsweetened almond milk

**Directions:**
1. Add all the ingredients except vegetables/fruits first
2. Blend until smooth
3. Add the vegetable/fruits
4. Blend until smooth
5. Add a few ice cubes and serve the smoothie
6. Enjoy!

**Nutrition Info:** Calories: 130; Fat: 9g; Carbohydrates: 15g; Protein: 3g

## Twisty Cucumber Honeydew

Servings: 2
Cooking Time: 5 Minutes
**Ingredients:**
- 1 cup ice
- 1 tablespoon fresh mint
- 2 cucumbers, chopped
- 1 cup honeydew melon, peeled, seeded, and chopped
- 1 cup coconut water

**Directions:**
1. Add all the ingredients except vegetables/fruits first
2. Blend until smooth
3. Add the vegetable/fruits
4. Blend until smooth
5. Add a few ice cubes and serve the smoothie
6. Enjoy!

**Nutrition Info:** Calories: 70; Fat: 1g; Carbohydrates: 13g; Protein: 2g

## Cocoa Pumpkin

Servings: 2
Cooking Time: 5 Minutes
**Ingredients:**
- ¼ teaspoon pumpkin spice
- 1 tablespoon maple syrup
- 2 tablespoons organic unsweetened cocoa powder
- ¼ frozen banana, sliced
- ½ Barlett pear, cored
- 3 cups baby spinach
- 1 cup organic pumpkin puree
- 1 cup unsweetened almond milk

**Directions:**
1. Add all the ingredients except vegetables/fruits first
2. Blend until smooth
3. Add the vegetable/fruits
4. Blend until smooth
5. Add a few ice cubes and serve the smoothie
6. Enjoy!

**Nutrition Info:** Calories: 486; Fat: 28g; Carbohydrates: 64g; Protein: 11g

## Lemon-lettuce Cooler

Servings: 2
Cooking Time: 5 Minutes
**Ingredients:**
- 1 green cucumber, deseeded and chopped
- 1 green apple, cored and quartered
- A handful of romaine lettuce, chopped
- 1 small head of broccoli, chopped
- A handful of kale stems re moved
- 3-4 celery stalk, chopped
- 1 teaspoon freshly squeezed lemon juice
- 3-4 ice cubes (optional)

**Directions:**

1. Combine all the ingredients in your blender and whizz it on high for 30 seconds.
**Nutrition Info:** (Per Serving): Calories- 128, Fat- 0 g, Protein- 7.2 g, Carbohydrates- 49 g


## Avocado Detox Smoothie

Servings: 3
Cooking Time: 10 Minutes
**Ingredients:**
- 4 cups spinach, chopped
- 1 avocado, chopped
- 3 cups apple juice
- 2 apples, unpeeled, cored and chopped

**Directions:**
1. Add all the listed ingredients to a blender
2. Blend until you have a smooth and creamy texture
3. Serve chilled and enjoy!

**Nutrition Info:** Calories: 336; Fat: 13.8g; Carbohydrates: 55.8g; Protein: 3g


## Apple-broccoli Smoothie

Servings: 2
Cooking Time: 5 Minutes
**Ingredients:**
- 1 ½ cup freshly squeezed pineapple juice
- 1 cup baby spinach
- 1 cup broccoli florets
- ½ green pear, cored and chopped
- ½ apple, cored and chopped
- ½ avocado, peeled and chopped
- ½ teaspoon lemon juice

**Directions:**
1. Whizz up all the ingredients u the blender for 30 seconds and enjoy.

**Nutrition Info:** (Per Serving): Calories- 379, Fat- 9.3 g, Protein- 15 g, Carbohydrates- 71 g


## Hearty Cucumber Quencher

Servings: 2
Cooking Time: 5 Minutes
**Ingredients:**
- 2 cups kale, chopped
- 1 fuji apple, quartered
- 1 large cucumber, cubed

**Directions:**
1. Add all the ingredients except vegetables/fruits first
2. Blend until smooth
3. Add the vegetable/fruits
4. Blend until smooth
5. Add a few ice cubes and serve the smoothie
6. Enjoy!

**Nutrition Info:** Calories: 180; Fat: 2g; Carbohydrates: 40g; Protein: 5g


## Mango Pepper Smoothie

Servings: 2
Cooking Time: 5 Minutes
**Ingredients:**

- 2 cups fresh coconut water
- 2 cups mango, peeled and chopped
- ¼ cup freshly squeezed lime juice
- A pinch of cayenne pepper
- 1-2 cubes of ice

**Directions:**
1. Place all the ingredients into the blender and pulse on high for 30 seconds or until the smoothie has reached your desired consistency.

**Nutrition Info:** (Per Serving): Calories-160, Fat- 0 g, Protein- 3 g, Carbohydrates- 40 g

## Honeydewmelon And Mint Blast

Servings: 2
Cooking Time: 2 Minutes
**Ingredients:**
- Cup cucumber, peeled and chopped
- 1 cup honeydew melon, peeled and chopped
- 1 cup freshly squeezed pear juice
- ¼ cup freshly squeezed lime juice
- ¼ cup fresh mint leaves, washed
- 2-3 cubes of ice (optional)

**Directions:**
1. Place all the ingredients into your blender and puree until smooth.

**Nutrition Info:** (Per Serving): Calories- 134, Fat-0 g, Protein- 2 g, Carbohydrates-33 g

## Apple And Green Slush

Servings: 1
Cooking Time: 2 Minutes
**Ingredients:**
- 1 granny smith apple, cored and chopped
- 1 large, ripe banana, chopped (fresh or frozen)
- ½ cup Italian flat leaf parsley
- 1 cup collard greens (stems removed)
- 1 teaspoon freshly squeezed lemon juice
- A few cubes of ice

**Directions:**
1. Add all the ingredients to your blender and blend until smooth.

**Nutrition Info:** (Per Serving): Calories- 105, Fat- 0 g, Protein- 2 g, Carbohydrates-26 g

## Apple And Pear Detox Wonder

Servings: 2
Cooking Time: 5 Minutes
**Ingredients:**
- 1 apple, cored and chopped
- 1 pear, cored and chopped
- 1 cup kale leaves, washed and stems removed
- 1 cup dandelion greens, washed
- ½ cup arugula, washed
- 1/2 cup freshly squeezed lemon juice
- 1 cup filtered water
- ½ teaspoon freshly grated ginger
- ½ teaspoon of cayenne pepper powder
- 1 teaspoon of raw organic honey (optional)
- 1 teaspoon Maca powder

**Directions:**

1.  Load your blender with all the above ingredients and blend until rich and creamy.
**Nutrition Info:** (Per Serving): Calories- 260, Fat- 2 g, Protein- 4 g, Carbohydrates- 67 g

## Very-berry Orange

Servings: 1 Large
Cooking Time: 2 Minutes
**Ingredients:**
- 1 cup blueberries, fresh or frozen
- 1 cup raspberries, fresh or frozen
- 2 large oranges, peeled and chopped
- A few ice cubes

**Directions:**
1.  Add everything to the blender and process on high for 30 seconds.
2.  Pour into glass and serve chilled.
**Nutrition Info:** (Per Serving): Calories- 132, Fat-0 g, Protein- 2 g, Carbohydrates- 34 g

## Lime And Lemon Detox Punch

Servings: 2
Cooking Time: 5 Minutes
**Ingredients:**
- 1 banana, chopped (fresh or frozen)
- ½ cup blueberries (fresh or frozen)
- 1 cup fresh kale stems chopped off
- ½ sweet lime, peeled, de-seeded and chopped
- 1 tablespoon freshly squeezed Lemon juice
- ½ tablespoon freshly grated ginger
- 1 cup filtered water
- 1 teaspoon raw organic honey
- A pinch of Celtic salt

**Directions:**
1.  Place all the ingredients into your blender and puree it on medium high until the smoothie is thick and frothy.
**Nutrition Info:** (Per Serving): Calories- 190, Fat- 1 g, Protein- 3 g, Carbohydrates- 51 g

## Dandellion- Orange Smoothie

Servings: 2
Cooking Time: 5 Minutes
**Ingredients:**
- 1 cup unsweetened almond milk
- 1 cup dandelion greens, washed and chopped
- 1 cup kale, (stems removed)
- 1 large orange, peeled and de seeded
- ½ lime, peeled and deseeded
- 1 ripe banana (fresh or frozen)
- ¼ teaspoon freshly grated ginger
- 1 tablespoon Chia seeds (soaked)
- 2-3 ice cubes

**Directions:**
1.  Add all the ingredients to your blender and process until smooth and creamy.
**Nutrition Info:** (Per Serving): Calories- 320, Fat- 4 g, Protein- 9 g, Carbohydrates- 64 g

# PROTEIN SMOOTHIES

## Glorious Cinnamon Roll Smoothie

Servings: 1
Cooking Time: 10 Minutes
**Ingredients:**
- 1 cup unsweetened almond milk
- ½ teaspoon cinnamon
- ¼ teaspoon vanilla extract
- 1 tablespoon chia seeds
- 2 tablespoons vanilla protein powder
- 1 cup ice cubs

**Directions:**
1. Add all the listed ingredients into your blender
2. Blend until smooth
3. Serve chilled and enjoy!

**Nutrition Info:** Calories: 145; Fat: 4g; Carbohydrates: 1.6g; Protein: 0.6g

## The Great Avocado And Almond Delight

Servings: 1
Cooking Time: 10 Minutes
**Ingredients:**
- ½ avocado, peeled, pitted and sliced
- ½ cup almond milk, vanilla and unsweetened
- ½ teaspoon vanilla extract
- ½ cup half and half
- 1 tablespoon almond butter
- 1 scoop Zero Carb protein powder
- Pinch of cinnamon
- 2-4 ice cubes
- Liquid stevia

**Directions:**
1. Add all the listed ingredients into your blender
2. Blend until smooth
3. Serve chilled and enjoy!

**Nutrition Info:** Calories: 252; Fat: 18g; Carbohydrates: 5g; Protein: 17g

## Healthy Chocolate Milkshake

Servings: 2
Cooking Time: 10 Minutes
**Ingredients:**
- 1 Scoop Whey isolate chocolate protein powder
- 16 ounces unsweetened almond milk, vanilla
- 1 pack stevia
- ½ cup crushed ice

**Directions:**
1. Add all the listed ingredients to a blender
2. Blend until you have a smooth and creamy texture
3. Serve chilled and enjoy!

**Nutrition Info:** Calories: 292; Fat: 25g; Carbohydrates: 4g; Protein: 15g

# Apple Mango Cucumber Crush

Servings: 3
Cooking Time: 5 Minutes
**Ingredients:**
- ½ cup freshly pressed red grapefruit juice
- 1 cup fresh kale, stems removed and chopped
- 1 large apple, cored and chopped
- ½ cup mango, peeled and chopped
- 1 cup English cucumber, chopped
- 1-2 small stalks of celery, chopped
- 5 teaspoons of hemp seeds
- 1 tablespoon pure coconut oil
- 3 -4 teaspoons of fresh mint leaves, chopped
- 4-5 ice cubes

**Directions:**
1. Add all the above listed items into the blender and blend until well combined.

**Nutrition Info:** (Per Serving): Calories- 265, Fat- 13 g, Protein- 10 g, Carbohydrates- 33 g

# Blueberry And Avocado Smoothie

Servings: 1
Cooking Time: 10 Minutes
**Ingredients:**
- 1/4 cup frozen blueberries, unsweetened
- ½ avocado, peeled, pitted and sliced
- 1 cup unsweetened milk, vanilla
- 1 scoop coconut Zero Carb protein powder
- 1 tablespoon heavy cream
- Liquid stevia

**Directions:**
1. Add all the listed ingredients into your blender
2. Blend until smooth
3. Serve chilled and enjoy!

**Nutrition Info:** Calories: 372; Fat: 22g; Carbohydrates: 4g; Protein: 32g

# Mad Mocha Glass

Servings: 2
Cooking Time: 5 Minutes
**Ingredients:**
- 4 ice cubes
- 1 scoop 100% chocolate whey protein
- ½ scoop vanilla protein powder
- 6 ounces water
- 6 ounces cold coffee

**Directions:**
1. Add all the ingredients except vegetables/fruits first
2. Blend until smooth
3. Add the vegetable/fruits
4. Blend until smooth
5. Add a few ice cubes and serve the smoothie
6. Enjoy!

**Nutrition Info:** Calories: 306; Fat: 4g; Carbohydrates: 43g; Protein: 28g

## Pineapple Protein Smoothie

Servings: 3-4
Cooking Time: 5 Minutes
**Ingredients:**
- 1 ½ cups pineapple, chopped
- 1 medium ripe banana, chopped
- 1 cup plain low fat yogurt
- 1 cup plain unsweetened almond milk
- 2-3 ice cubes

**Directions:**
1. Place everything in the blender jar, secure the lid and pulse until smooth.

**Nutrition Info:** (Per Serving): Calories- 170, Fat- 4.7 g, Protein- 11 g, Carbohydrates- 25 g

## Oat "n" Nut Breakfast Blend

Servings: 1 Large
Cooking Time: 5 Minutes
**Ingredients:**
- ½ cup unsweetened almond or soy milk
- ¼ cup rolled oats
- 1 large banana, chopped
- 3 teaspoons peanut butter
- ½ teaspoon raw organic honey

**Directions:**
1. Place all the ingredients into your blender and whirr it on high for 20 seconds or until the desired consistency has been reached. Pour into glasses and serve immediately.

**Nutrition Info:** (Per Serving): Calories- 330, Fat-20 g, Protein- 15 g, Carbohydrates- 28 g

## The Cacao Super Smoothie

Servings: 1
Cooking Time: 10 Minutes
**Ingredients:**
- ½ avocado, peeled, pitted, sliced
- ½ cup frozen blueberries, unsweetened
- ½ cup almond milk, vanilla, unsweetened
- ½ cup half and half
- 1 scoop whey vanilla protein powder
- 1 tablespoon cacao powder
- Liquid stevia

**Directions:**
1. Add listed ingredients to a blender
2. Blend until you get a smooth and creamy texture
3. Serve chilled and enjoy!

**Nutrition Info:** Calories: 445; Fat: 14g; Carbohydrates: 9g; Protein: 16g

## Snicker Doodle Smoothie

Servings: 2 Small
Cooking Time: 2 Minutes
**Ingredients:**
- 1 cup unsweetened almond milk
- 1 teaspoon raw, organic cacao powder
- 1/3 cup peanut butter or peanut powder

- 1 large ripe banana, chopped
- 3-5 ice cubes

**Directions:**
1. Whizz all the ingredients in the blender until smooth and serve.

**Nutrition Info:** (Per Serving): Calories- 315, Fat- 10 g, Protein- 28 g, Carbohydrates-45 g

## Green Protein Smoothie

Servings: 2
Cooking Time: 10 Minutes
**Ingredients:**
- 2 bananas
- 4 cups mixed greens
- 2 tablespoons almond butter
- 1 cup almond milk, unsweetened

**Directions:**
1. Add all the listed ingredients to a blender
2. Blend until you have a smooth and creamy texture
3. Serve chilled and enjoy!

**Nutrition Info:** Calories: 230; Fat: 5.8g; Carbohydrates: 39.5g; Protein: 7.8g

## Sweet Protein And Cherry Shake

Servings: 2
Cooking Time: 5 Minutes
**Ingredients:**
- 1 cup water
- 3 cups spinach
- 2 bananas, sliced
- 2 cups frozen cherries
- 2 tablespoons cacao powder
- 4 tablespoons hemp seeds, shelled

**Directions:**
1. Add all the ingredients except vegetables/fruits first
2. Blend until smooth
3. Add the vegetable/fruits
4. Blend until smooth
5. Add a few ice cubes and serve the smoothie
6. Enjoy!

**Nutrition Info:** Calories: 111; Fat: 3g; Carbohydrates: 9g; Protein: 13g

## Protein-packed Root Beer Shake

Servings: 2
Cooking Time: 5 Minutes
**Ingredients:**
- ½ cup fat-free vanilla yogurt
- 1 scoop vanilla whey protein
- 1½ cups root beet
- 1 scoop vanilla casein protein

**Directions:**
1. Add all the ingredients except vegetables/fruits first
2. Blend until smooth
3. Add the vegetable/fruits
4. Blend until smooth
5. Add a few ice cubes and serve the smoothie
6. Enjoy!

**Nutrition Info:** Calories: 677; Fat: 56g; Carbohydrates: 39g; Protein: 16g

## Strawberry Coconut Snowflake

Servings: 2
Cooking Time: 2 Minutes
**Ingredients:**
- ½ unsweetened, fresh coconut milk
- 1 cup whole strawberries (fresh or frozen)
- ½ cup plain low fat Greek yogurt
- ¼ cup freshly squeezed orange
- ½ teaspoon raw organic honey
- 2-3 ice cubes

**Directions:**
1. Just place all the ingredients into the blender and pulse until smooth. Serve immediately!

**Nutrition Info:** (Per Serving): Calories- 160, Fat- 2.8 g, Protein- 12 g, Carbohydrates- 24 g

## Raspberry And White Chocolate Shake

Servings: 2
Cooking Time: 5 Minutes
**Ingredients:**
- 2 scoops whey vanilla protein powder
- 1 tablespoon chia seeds
- 1 tablespoon white chocolate chips
- 2 tablespoons water
- 1 cup coconut milk, unsweetened
- ¾ cup frozen raspberries

**Directions:**
1. Add all the ingredients except vegetables/fruits first
2. Blend until smooth
3. Add the vegetable/fruits
4. Blend until smooth
5. Add a few ice cubes and serve the smoothie
6. Enjoy!

**Nutrition Info:** Calories: 574; Fat: 35g; Carbohydrates: 34g; Protein: 34g

## Berry Orange Madness

Servings: 2-3
Cooking Time: 2 Minutes
**Ingredients:**
- 1 cup mixed berries (fresh or frozen)
- 1 large orange, peeled, seeded and segmented
- 1 cup low fat plain yogurt
- 1 banana, chopped (frozen)
- ¼ teaspoon vanilla extract
- 1-2 ice cubes

**Directions:**
1. Pour all the ingredients into your blender and process until smooth.

**Nutrition Info:** (Per Serving): Calories-210, Fat-2 g, Protein- 8.3 g, Carbohydrates- 40 g

# WEIGHT LOSS SMOOTHIES

## Banana And Spinach Raspberry Smoothie

Servings: 2
Cooking Time: 5 Minutes
**Ingredients:**
- 1 tablespoons cilantro
- 1 cup crushed ice
- 1 tablespoon ground flaxseed
- ½ cup raspberries
- 2 dates
- 2 bananas
- 1 cup spinach, chopped

**Directions:**
1. Add all the ingredients except vegetables/fruits first
2. Blend until smooth
3. Add the vegetable/fruits
4. Blend until smooth
5. Add a few ice cubes and serve the smoothie
6. Enjoy!

**Nutrition Info:** Calories: 120; Fat: 2g; Carbohydrates: 30g; Protein: 3g

## Apple Broccoli Smoothie

Servings: 2
Cooking Time: 5 Minutes
**Ingredients:**
- 1 tablespoon seaweed, crushed
- 1 cup ice, crushed
- 1 stalk celery, diced
- 1 tablespoon cilantro, chopped
- 1 cup broccoli, diced
- 1 apple, quartered

**Directions:**
1. Add all the ingredients except vegetables/fruits first
2. Blend until smooth
3. Add the vegetable/fruits
4. Blend until smooth
5. Add a few ice cubes and serve the smoothie
6. Enjoy!

**Nutrition Info:** Calories: 223; Fat: 1g; Carbohydrates: 51g; Protein: 9g

## Coconutty Apple Smoothie

Servings: 1
Cooking Time: 2 Minutes
**Ingredients:**
- 1 cup apple, cored and chopped
- ½ cup organic coconut milk
- 1 small banana, chopped
- 2 teaspoons almond butter
- ½ cup kale, chopped
- 1 ½ teaspoon flaxseed powder
- ½ teaspoon cinnamon powder

**Directions:**
1.   Combine all the ingredients together in the blender and pulse for 30 seconds. Pour into a glass and enjoy.
**Nutrition Info:** (Per Serving): Calories- 330, Fat- 14 g, Protein- 5.8 g, Carbohydrates- 51 g

## Raspberry- Grapefruit Smoothie

Servings: 2-3
Cooking Time: 5 Minutes
**Ingredients:**
- 2 cups fresh spinach, chopped
- ½ grapefruits, peeled and de seeded
- ½ cup raspberries (fresh or frozen)
- 1 California orange, peeled and de seeded
- ¼ cup whole strawberries (fresh or frozen)
- 1 tablespoon Chia seeds, soaked
- 1 ½ cups of filtered water

**Directions:**
1.   To your blender, add all the items listed above and blend until smooth and creamy.
**Nutrition Info:** (Per Serving): Calories- 164, Fat- 5.5 g, Protein- 5.6 g, Carbohydrates- 29 g

## Sunrise Smoothie

Servings: 1 Large
Cooking Time: 2 Minutes
**Ingredients:**
- 1 cup mango, chopped (fresh or frozen)
- ¼ cup avocado, chopped
- 1 cup plain yogurt
- ¼ teaspoon vanilla essence
- 1 tablespoon freshly squeezed lemon juice
- 1 teaspoon raw, organic honey
- A handful of ice cubes

**Directions:**
1.   Place the ingredients into the blender and secure the lid tightly. Run the blender on high for 25 seconds and serve chilled.
**Nutrition Info:** (Per Serving): Calories-300, Fat-9 g, Protein- 5 g, Carbohydrates- 56 g

## Spiced Pineapple Smoothie

Servings: 2
Cooking Time: 5 Minutes
**Ingredients:**
- 1 cup pineapple, chopped (fresh or frozen)
- 1 large banana, chopped
- 2 tablespoons freshly squeezed lemon juice
- 1 teaspoon freshly grated ginger
- 1 tablespoon maca powder
- 1 tablespoon flax seed powder
- ¼ teaspoon cayenne pepper
- 1 ¼ cup filtered water

**Directions:**
1.   Pour all the ingredients into the blender and process it for 45 seconds on medium speed and serve.
**Nutrition Info:** (Per Serving): Calories- 255, Fat- 3.8 g, Protein- 4.5 g, Carbohydrates- 57 g

# Flax And Kiwi Spinach Smoothie

Servings: 2
Cooking Time: 5 Minutes
**Ingredients:**
- 1 cup crushed ice
- 3 tablespoons ground flax
- 3 kiwis, diced
- 1 stalk celery, chopped
- 1 banana, chopped
- 2 apples, quartered
- 1 cup spinach, chopped

**Directions:**
1. Add all the ingredients except vegetables/fruits first
2. Blend until smooth
3. Add the vegetable/fruits
4. Blend until smooth
5. Add a few ice cubes and serve the smoothie
6. Enjoy!

**Nutrition Info:** Calories: 142; Fat: 7g; Carbohydrates: 16g; Protein: 6g

# Meanie-greenie Weigh Loss Smoothie

Servings: 2-3
Cooking Time: 5 Minutes
**Ingredients:**
- 1 cup kale, stems removed
- 1 cup green cucumber, de-seeded and chopped
- 1 celery stalk, chopped
- 1 small pear, peeled, cored and chopped
- 1 teaspoon freshly grated ginger
- A handful of parsley
- 1 ½ cups of filtered water
- 1 teaspoon freshly squeezed lemon juice

**Directions:**
1. Place all the ingredients in the order listed above and pulse until the desired consistency is attained.

**Nutrition Info:** (Per Serving): Calories- 64.3, Fat- 0.3 g, Protein- 1 g, Carbohydrates- 15.8 g

# Kale Celery Smoothie

Servings: 2
Cooking Time: 10 Minutes
**Ingredients:**
- 3 cups kale, chopped
- 2 stalks celery, diced
- 1 red apple, cored and diced
- 2 cups almond milk, unsweetened
- 1 ¼ cups ice
- 2 teaspoons honey
- 2 tablespoons flaxseed, ground

**Directions:**
1. Add all the listed ingredients to a blender
2. Blend until you have a smooth and creamy texture
3. Serve chilled and enjoy!

**Nutrition Info:** Calories: 341; Fat: 29.8g; Carbohydrates: 18.6g; Protein: 5.3g

## Carrot Spice Smoothie

Servings: 2
Cooking Time: 5 Minutes
**Ingredients:**
- 1 cup unsweetened almond milk
- 1 ripe banana, chopped
- 1 cup carrots, peeled and chopped
- 4 ounces plain yogurt
- 1 tablespoon raw organic honey
- ¼ teaspoon freshly grated ginger
- ¼ teaspoon cinnamon powder
- A pinch of nutmeg powder
- 3-4 ice cubes

**Directions:**
1. Add all the ingredients into the blender one by one and pulse until thick and creamy.

**Nutrition Info:** (Per Serving): Calories- 295, Fat- 3.5 g, Protein- 9 g, Carbohydrates- 61.5 g


## Zucchini Apple Smoothie

Servings: 2
Cooking Time: 5 Minutes
**Ingredients:**
- 1½ cups crushed ice
- 1 tablespoon Spirulina
- 1 lemon, juiced
- 1 stalk celery
- ¾ avocado
- 2 apples, quartered
- ½ cup zucchini, diced

**Directions:**
1. Add all the ingredients except vegetables/fruits first
2. Blend until smooth
3. Add the vegetable/fruits
4. Blend until smooth
5. Add a few ice cubes and serve the smoothie
6. Enjoy!

**Nutrition Info:** Calories: 80; Fat: 4g; Carbohydrates: 11g; Protein: 2g


## Straight Up Avocado And Kale Smoothie

Servings: 2
Cooking Time: 5 Minutes
**Ingredients:**
- 1 tablespoon spirulina
- 1 cup chamomile tea
- 1 tablespoon Chia seeds
- 1 stalk celery
- 1 cup cucumber
- ½ avocado, diced
- 1 cup kale, chopped

**Directions:**
1. Add all the ingredients except vegetables/fruits first

2. Blend until smooth
3. Add the vegetable/fruits
4. Blend until smooth
5. Add a few ice cubes and serve the smoothie
6. Enjoy!

**Nutrition Info:** Calories: 236; Fat: 6g; Carbohydrates: 46g; Protein: 4g

## Berry-banana-spinach Smoothie

Servings: 2
Cooking Time: 5 Minutes
**Ingredients:**
- 1 cup mixed berries (fresh or frozen)
- 1 cup baby spinach, washed and chopped
- ½ large banana, chopped (fresh r frozen)
- 1 teaspoon coconut oil
- 1 tablespoon flax seeds
- ¼ teaspoon cayenne pepper powder
- 1 cup filtered water

**Directions:**
1. Place all the ingredients in the blender and run I on high for 30 seconds or until the desired consistency is got.

**Nutrition Info:** (Per Serving): Calories- 250, Fat-14 g, Protein-3 g, Carbohydrates-33 g

## Healthy Raspberry And Coconut Glass

Servings: 1
Cooking Time: 10 Minutes
**Ingredients:**
- ¼ cup raspberries
- 1 tablespoon pepitas
- 1 tablespoon coconut oil
- ½ cup of coconut milk
- 1 cup 50/50 salad mix
- 1 ½ cups of water
- 1 pack stevia

**Directions:**
1. Add listed ingredients to a blender
2. Blend until you have a smooth and creamy texture
3. Serve chilled and enjoy!

**Nutrition Info:** Calories: 408; Fat: 41g; Carbohydrates: 10g; Protein: 5g

## Peanut Butter Berry Smoothie

Servings: 2
Cooking Time: 2 Minutes
**Ingredients:**
- 1 tablespoon peanut butter
- 2 cups strawberry (fresh or frozen)
- 1 large banana, chopped (fresh or frozen)
- ½ cup plain or Greek yogurt
- A handful of ice cubes

**Directions:**
1. Add all the ingredients into the blender and whip it up until smooth and nice.

2. Pour into cool serving glasses and enjoy.
**Nutrition Info:** (Per Serving): Calories- 327, Fat- 7 g, Protein- 18 g, Carbohydrates- 55 g

## Carrot Coconut Smoothie

Servings: 2
Cooking Time: 5 Minutes
**Ingredients:**
- 6 ounces carrots, chopped
- 1 orange, peeled
- 4 ounces pineapple
- 1 teaspoon Camu Camu
- 2 tablespoons coconut flakes
- 1 cup ice
- 1 cup of water

**Directions:**
1. Add all the listed ingredients to a blender
2. Blend until you have a smooth and creamy texture
3. Serve chilled and enjoy!
**Nutrition Info:** Calories: 140; Fat: 2g; Carbohydrates: 29g; Protein: 2g

# KID FRIENDLY HEALTHY SMOOTHIES

## Grape- Lettuce Chiller

Servings: 2
Cooking Time: 2 Minutes
**Ingredients:**
- 1 cup green grapes, seedless
- 1 large cup romaine lettuce, washed and chopped
- ½ large apple, cored and chopped
- 2-3 teaspoons freshly squeezed lemon juice
- ½ teaspoon raw organic honey
- 4-5 ice cubes

**Directions:**
1. To you blender, add the above ingredient and pulse until smooth.

**Nutrition Info:** (Per Serving): Calories-82, Fat- 0 g, Protein- 1.4 g , Carbohydrates- 22 g

## Pineapple Papaya Perfection Smoothie

Servings: 3
Cooking Time: 5 Minutes
**Ingredients:**
- 2 cups papaya. Peeled and chopped
- 1 cup plain low fat yogurt
- ½ cup pineapple, peeled and chopped
- 1 teaspoon grated coconut
- 1 teaspoon flax seed powder
- 2 teaspoon freshly squeezed lemon juice
- 4-5 ice cubes

**Directions:**
1. To make this smoothie, place everything into the blender and pulse until smooth. Serve immediately.

**Nutrition Info:** (Per Serving): Calories- 230, Fat- 1.4 g, Protein- 12.5 g, Carbohydrates- 65 g

## Carrot Peach Blush

Servings: 2-3
Cooking Time: 5 Minutes
**Ingredients:**
- 1 cup unsweetened almond milk
- 1 ripe banana, chopped
- 2 large peaches, pitted and chopped
- 1 large carrot, peeled and chopped
- 1 teaspoon freshly grated ginger
- 3-4 ice cubes

**Directions:**
1. To your high speed blender, add all the above mentioned items and process on high for 30 seconds. Pour into serving glasses and enjoy immediately.

**Nutrition Info:** (Per Serving): Calories- 110, Fat- 5 g, Protein- 2 g, Carbohydrates- 15 g

## Chilled Watermelon Krush

Servings: 2
Cooking Time: 2 Minutes
**Ingredients:**
- 2 cups watermelon, chopped (seedless)

- 5-6 fresh mint leaves, roughly torn
- ½ cup low fat, plain yogurt
- 1 ½ teaspoons raw organic honey
- 3-4 ice cubes

**Directions:**
1. Add all the above ingredients into your blender jar and pulse until thick and frothy.

**Nutrition Info:** (Per Serving): Calories- 185, Fat- 0 g, Protein- 13 g, Carbohydrates- 35 g

## Minty Chocolate Smoothie

Servings: 3
Cooking Time: 10 Minutes
**Ingredients:**
- 4 tablespoons cocoa powder
- 2 cups almond milk
- 2 bananas, frozen
- 1 2/3 cups spinach leaves
- ½ cup mint leaves
- Stevia liquid, to taste

**Directions:**
1. Add all the listed ingredients to a blender
2. Blend until you have a smooth and creamy texture
3. Serve chilled and enjoy!

**Nutrition Info:** Calories: 352; Fat: 29.7g; Carbohydrates: 25.3g; Protein: 5.2g

## Peanut Butter Broccoli Smoothie

Servings: 3
Cooking Time: 5 Minutes
**Ingredients:**
- 1 cup unsweetened almond milk
- 1 cup fresh spinach, washed and chopped
- 1 cup broccoli florets, washed and chopped
- 1 large kale leaf, washed and chopped
- 1 ripe banana, chopped
- 2 teaspoons peanut butter
- 1 teaspoon raw organic honey (optional)

**Directions:**
1. Add all the ingredients into the high speed blender and whizz until smooth.

**Nutrition Info:** (Per Serving): Calories- 325, Fat- 14 g, Protein- 10 g, Carbohydrates- 46 g

## Delish Pineapple And Coconut Milk Smoothie

Servings: 2
Cooking Time: 5 Minutes
**Ingredients:**
- ¾ cup of coconut water
- ¼ cup pineapple, frozen

**Directions:**
1. Add listed ingredients to a blender
2. Blend on high until you have a smooth and creamy texture
3. Serve chilled and enjoy!

**Nutrition Info:** Calories: 132; Fat: 12g; Carbohydrates: 7g; Protein: 1g

## Berry Almond Breakfast Blend

Servings: 2
Cooking Time: 2 Minutes
**Ingredients:**
- ½ cup fresh butter milk
- ½ cup plain low fat yogurt
- ¼ cup fresh raspberries
- ¼ cup seedless red grapes
- 1 small ripe banana, chopped
- ½ cup blueberries (fresh or frozen)
- 2 teaspoons rolled oats
- 1 teaspoon flaxseed powder
- 1/4 cup almonds

**Directions:**
1. Blend all the ingredients into the blender and enjoy!

**Nutrition Info:** (Per Serving): Calories-260, Fat- 6.2 g, Protein- 8.9 g, Carbohydrates- 45 g

## Blueberry Pineapple Blast Smoothie

Servings: 2
Cooking Time: 2 Minutes
**Ingredients:**
- 1 cup freshly squeezed pineapple juice
- 1/3 cup fresh, organic coconut milk
- 1 cup whole blueberries (fresh or frozen)
- 2 teaspoons of shredded coconut
- 3-4 ice cubes

**Directions:**
1. Add all the ingredients into the blender jar and pulse it on high for 30 seconds or until smooth.

**Nutrition Info:** (Per Serving): Calories- 265, Fat- 10 g, Protein- 3 g, Carbohydrates- 45 g

## The Blueberry And Chocolate Delight

Servings: 1
Cooking Time: 10 Minutes
**Ingredients:**
- ½ cup whole milk yogurt
- ¼ cup blackberries
- 1 pack stevia
- 1 tablespoon MCT oil
- 1 tablespoon Dutch Processed Cocoa Powder
- 2 tablespoons Macadamia nuts, chopped
- 1½ cups water

**Directions:**
1. Add all the ingredients except vegetables/fruits first
2. Blend until smooth
3. Add the vegetable/fruits
4. Blend until smooth
5. Add a few ice cubes and serve the smoothie
6. Enjoy!

**Nutrition Info:** Calories: 175; Fat: 2g; Carbohydrates: 33g; Protein: 6g

# Maple Chocolate Smoothie

Servings: 2
Cooking Time: 10 Minutes
**Ingredients:**
- 4 tablespoons cocoa powder
- 2 ½ cups of almond milk
- 1 cup oats, rolled
- 1 teaspoon vanilla extract
- 1 tablespoon maple syrup
- 2 tablespoons almond butter

**Directions:**
1. Add all the listed ingredients to a blender
2. Blend until you have a smooth and creamy texture
3. Serve chilled and enjoy!

**Nutrition Info:** Calories: 170; Fat: 7.2g; Carbohydrates: 23.8g; Protein: 5.6g

# Very Berry Blueberry Wonder

Servings: 2
Cooking Time: 5 Minutes
**Ingredients:**
- ½ cup whole blueberries (fresh or frozen)
- 1 tangerine, peeled and seeded
- 1 medium beet, peeled and chopped
- ½ large banana, chopped (fresh or frozen)
- 1 tablespoons chia seed
- A large pinch of cinnamon powder
- 1/3 cup low fat plain yogurt
- 4-5 ice cubes

**Directions:**
1. Whizz up all the ingredients in a blender, pour into glass and serve!

**Nutrition Info:** (Per Serving): Calories-285, Fat- 4 g, Protein- 20 g, Carbohydrates- 50 g

# Raspberry Pecan Date Delight

Servings: 1 Large
Cooking Time: 2 Minutes
**Ingredients:**
- 1 ripe banana, chopped
- ½ cup whole raspberries (fresh or frozen)
- 1 teaspoon coconut oil
- 1 tablespoon pecan halves
- 1 date, pitted
- 1 teaspoon flaxseed powder
- 1 cup filtered water

**Directions:**
1. Pour all the ingredients into your blender and process until smooth.

**Nutrition Info:** (Per Serving): Calories- 375, Fat- 15 g, Protein- 3.5 g, Carbohydrates- 65 g

# Raw Chocolate Smoothie

Servings: 2
Cooking Time: 10 Minutes
**Ingredients:**

- 2 medium bananas
- 4 tablespoons peanut butter, raw
- 1 cup almond milk
- 3 tablespoons cocoa powder, raw
- 2 tablespoons honey, raw

**Directions:**
1. Add all the listed ingredients to a blender
2. Blend until you have a smooth and creamy texture
3. Serve chilled and enjoy!

**Nutrition Info:** Calories: 217; Fat: 2.8g; Carbohydrates: 52.7g; Protein: 3.4g

## Ultimate Berry Blush

Servings: 4
Cooking Time: 5 Minutes
**Ingredients:**
- 2 cups mixed berries (fresh or frozen)
- 2 cups low fat plain yogurt
- 2 large bananas, chopped (fresh r frozen0
- 1 teaspoon cashews
- 4-5 ice cubes

**Directions:**
1. Combine all the ingredients in a high speed blender and whirr until thick and smooth.

**Nutrition Info:** (Per Serving): Calories- 150, Fat- 1.5 g, Protein- 5 g, Carbohydrates- 30 g

## Date Pomegranate Wonder

Servings: 3
Cooking Time: 5 Minutes
**Ingredients:**
- 1 cup whole blueberries (fresh or frozen)
- 1 cup unsweetened, fresh coconut milk
- ½ cup baby spinach, washed and chopped
- ½ cup pomegranate seeds
- 5-6 dates, pitted
- 2 teaspoons Chia seeds, soaked
- 4-5 ice cubes (optional)

**Directions:**
1. Whizz up all the ingredients in a blender, pour into glass and serve!

**Nutrition Info:** (Per Serving): Calories- 525, Fat- 18 g, Protein- 7 g, Carbohydrates- 100 g

# HEART HEALTHY SMOOTHIES

## Pina Berry Smoothie

Servings: 2
Cooking Time: 2 Minutes
**Ingredients:**
- 1 cup whole strawberries (fresh or frozen)
- 1 cup pineapple, chopped fresh or frozen)
- 1 teaspoon vanilla extract
- 1 cup plain yogurt
- 4-5 ice cubes

**Directions:**
1. Pour everything into the blender and blend until thick and frothy.

**Nutrition Info:** (Per Serving): Calories: 12, Fat-0.5 g, Protein-6 g, Carbohydrates-25 g

## Vanilla- Mango Madness

Servings: 1
Cooking Time: 2 Minutes
**Ingredients:**
- 1 cup mango, chopped (fresh or frozen)
- 1 cup plain yogurt
- 1 tablespoon freshly squeezed lemon juice
- ¼ teaspoon vanilla extract
- ¼ teaspoon nutmeg powder
- 1 teaspoon raw organic honey
- A pinch of Celtic salt
- ¼ cup filtered water

**Directions:**
1. To your blender jar, add all the ingredients and whizz until thick and creamy.

**Nutrition Info:** (Per Serving): Calories- 160, Fat- 2 g, Protein- 7 g, Carbohydrates- 29.3 g

## Verry-berry Carrot Delight

Servings: 2
Cooking Time: 2 Minutes
**Ingredients:**
- 1 cup mixed berries
- ½ cup plain yogurt
- 1 cup almond milk
- 1 carrot, peeled and chopped
- A pinch or cinnamon powder

**Directions:**
1. Place all the ingredients in your blender and process it for 45 seconds.
2. Serve and enjoy immediately.

**Nutrition Info:** (Per Serving): Calories-159, Fat-3.5 g, Protein-8 g, Carbohydrates-24 g

## Cinn-apple Beet Smoothie

Servings: 1
Cooking Time: 2 Minutes
**Ingredients:**
- 1 large red beet, peeled and chopped
- 1 large carrot, peeled and chopped

- 1 red apple, cored and chopped
- 1 teaspoon freshly grated ginger
- 1 teaspoon cinnamon powder
- 1 teaspoon coconut oil
- ½ cup filtered water
- ½ teaspoon raw organic honey

**Directions:**
1. Load your blender with all the ingredients and process it on medium for 30 seconds and then on high speed for 45 seconds or until well combined.

**Nutrition Info:** (Per Serving): Calories- 211, Fat- 6 g, Protein- 11 g, Carbohydrates- 44 g

## Beet And Apple Smoothie

Servings: 2
Cooking Time: 5 Minutes
**Ingredients:**
- 2 beetroots, peeled and chopped
- ½ cup blueberries, fresh or frozen
- 1 apple, cored, peeled and chipped
- 1 teaspoon freshly grated ginger
- 1 cup filtered water

**Directions:**
1. Combine all the ingredients in the blender and pulse it on high for 1 minute or until smooth.

**Nutrition Info:** (Per Serving): Calories-88, Fat- 0 g, Protein- 2 g, Carbohydrates- 20 g

## Almond-banana Blend

Servings: 3
Cooking Time: 5 Minutes
**Ingredients:**
- 4 large, ripe bananas (fresh or frozen)
- 1 cup unsweetened almond milk
- 2 tablespoons almonds (soaked and chopped)
- 1 cup plain yogurt
- 3 teaspoons raw organic honey

**Directions:**
1. Pour all the ingredients into the blender and puree until a creamy smoothie is got.

**Nutrition Info:** (Per Serving): Calories- 192, Fat- 5 g, Protein- 5 g, Carbohydrates- 38 g

## Spinach And Grape Smoothie

Servings: 1 Large
Cooking Time: 5 Minutes
**Ingredients:**
- 1 cup red grapes (seedless)
- 2 cups baby spinach
- 1 banana (fresh or frozen)
- 1 tablespoon Chia seeds (soaked)
- 1 teaspoon freshly squeezed lemon juice
- A handful of ice cubes

**Directions:**
1. Load all the ingredients into your blender jar and secure it tightly with a lid.
2. Pulse it on medium speed for 30 seconds and on high for 1 minute or until smooth.

**Nutrition Info:** (Per Serving): Calories-107, Fat-2.4 g, Protein-1.5 g, Carbohydrates-26.5 g

## Melon And Soy Smoothie

Servings: 2
Cooking Time: 5 Minutes
**Ingredients:**
- 1 green cucumber, chopped
- 2 cups melon, chopped
- 1 ½ cups soybeans, boiled
- 4-5 fresh basil leaves
- 4-5 ice cubes

**Directions:**
1. Add all the ingredients into the blender and process it for 1 minute or until done.

**Nutrition Info:** (Per Serving): Calories- 200, Fat- 1.5 g, Protein- 10 g, Carbohydtaets-48 g

## Mint And Avocado Smoothie

Servings: 3
Cooking Time: 5 Minutes
**Ingredients:**
- 2 cups unsweetened almond milk
- 1 medium banana, chopped
- 2 cups of fresh spinach
- 1 kiwi, peeled and quartered
- Freshly squeezed juice of 1 lime
- 6-8 fresh mint leaves
- ½ avocado, pitted and chopped
- 1 teaspoon freshly grated ginger

**Directions:**
1. Place all the above listed ingredients in the same order into your blender jar and process it until thick and smooth.

**Nutrition Info:** (Per Serving): Calories- 254, Fat- 12 g, Protein-10 g, Carbohydrates- 31 g

## Chia-cacao Melon Smoothie

Servings: 2
Cooking Time: 5 Minutes
**Ingredients:**
- 1 cup fresh strawberries
- 1 cup cantaloupe, chopped
- 1 large banana (fresh or frozen)
- 2 large chard leaves, chopped
- 1 cup unsweetened almond milk
- 1 tablespoon cacao powder
- 1 tablespoons Chia seeds, soaked

**Directions:**
1. Pour all the ingredients into your blender and whizz it up on high speed for 45 seconds or until done.

**Nutrition Info:** (Per Serving): Calories- 330, Fat- 0 g, Protein- 11 g, Carbohydrates- 62 g

## Peach And Celery Smoothie

Servings: 2
Cooking Time: 5 Minutes

**Ingredients:**
- ½ green cucumber, chopped with peel on
- 1 large peach, pitted and chopped
- 1 orange, peeled and de seeded
- 2 tablespoons avocado flesh
- 2-3 stalks celery, washed and chopped
- 2 cups fresh Swiss chard, chopped
- ¾ cup filtered water
- 3-4 cubes of ice

**Directions:**
1. Combine all the above ingredients in your blender and process until the desired consistency is obtained.

**Nutrition Info:** (Per Serving): Calories- 255, Fat- 0 g, Protein- 8 g, Carbohydrates- 50 g

## Oatmeal Banana Smoothie

Servings: 2 Small
Cooking Time: 5 Minutes

**Ingredients:**
- 1 large banana (fresh or frozen)
- 1 persimmon, peeled and chopped
- 1 cup mango, chopped (fresh or frozen)
- 4 tablespoons rolled oats, soaked
- 1 tablespoon raw organic honey
- A pinch of cinnamon powder

**Directions:**
1. Place all the ingredients into the blender and blend until creamy.

**Nutrition Info:** (Per Serving): Calories- 420, Fat- 2 g, Protein- 9 g, Carbohydrates- 95 g

## Mango-ginger Tango

Servings: 2
Cooking Time: 5 Minutes

**Ingredients:**
- 1 cup pineapple, peeled and chopped
- 1 cup mango, chopped
- 1 large orange, peeled and de seeded
- ½ cup filtered water
- 2 cups fresh kale, stems removed and chopped
- 1 teaspoon freshly grated ginger
- 2-3 cubes of ice

**Directions:**
1. Place all the ingredients into the blended one by one and pulse until smooth.

**Nutrition Info:** (Per Serving): Calories- 355, Fat- 0 g, Protein- 9 g, Carbohydrates- 88 g

## Peach-ban-illa Smoothie

Servings: 2 Small
Cooking Time: 5 Minutes

**Ingredients:**
- 1 ¼ cup peaches, pitted and chopped
- 1 large banana (fresh or frozen)
- 1 cup plain yogurt
- 1 teaspoon vanilla extract
- 1 teaspoon Chia seeds, soaked

- A handful of ice

**Directions:**

1. Combine all the ingredients in the blender and blend until the desired consistency is got.

**Nutrition Info:** (Per Serving): Calories- 170, Fat- 2 g, Protein- 5 g, Carbohydrates- 45 g

## Hemp-avocado Smoothie

Servings: 2
Cooking Time: 5 Minutes

**Ingredients:**

- A red apple, cored and chopped
- 1 tablespoon avocado flesh
- 1 cup unsweetened almond milk
- 2 tablespoon hemp seeds
- 2 cups fresh baby spinach

**Directions:**

1. Pour all the ingredients into your blender and run in on high for 1 minute. Pour into tall glasses and enjoy!

**Nutrition Info:** (Per Serving): Calories- 350, Fat- 0 g, Protein- 10 g, Carbohydrates- 43 g

## Berry Banana Smoothie

Servings: 1
Cooking Time: 5 Minutes

**Ingredients:**

- 1 large orange, peeled and chopped
- 2 cups of mixed greens or baby spinach, washed
- 1 cup mixed berries (fresh or frozen)
- 1 banana, peeled and chopped
- 1-2 tablespoons avocado flesh
- 1 tablespoon of flax seeds, powdered
- 1 cup filtered water

**Directions:**

1. First add the liquids and the fruits to your blender, next add the greens and flax seeds and sauce the lid.
2. Process for 30 seconds on high or until the smoothie is thick and creamy.

**Nutrition Info:** (Per Serving): Calories- 334, Fat-8 g, Protein- 6 g, Carbohydrates- 65 g

# OVERALL HEALTH AND WELLNESS SMOOTHIES

## Nutty Berry Broccoli Smoothie

Servings: 3
Cooking Time: 5 Minutes
**Ingredients:**
- 2 bananas, chopped
- 1 ½ cup plain low fat yogurt
- ¼ cup filtered water
- 1 cup whole strawberries (fresh or frozen)
- ½ cup broccoli florets
- 1 tablespoon peanut butter
- 4-5 ice cubes

**Directions:**
1. Whizz all the ingredients in the blender until smooth and serve.

**Nutrition Info:** (Per Serving): Calories- 330, Fat- 4.8 g, Protein- 23 g, Carbohydrates-54 g

## Drink Your Salad Smoothie

Servings: 2
Cooking Time: 5 Minutes
**Ingredients:**
- 4 vine tomatoes, washed
- 1 teaspoon avocado flesh
- 1 red bell pepper, deseeded
- ½ green zucchini, chopped
- 3-4 celery stalks, chopped
- ¼ white onion
- 1 teaspoon of flax seed powder
- A pinch of cayenne pepper
- A pinch of paprika or chili powder
- ¼ cup filtered water

**Directions:**
1. Dump all the ingredients into the blender and whip it up until the smoothie is thick and creamy.

**Nutrition Info:** (Per Serving): Calories-458, Fat- 16.5 g, Protein- 16.8 g, Carbohydrates- 78 g

## Dragon- Berry Smoothie

Servings: 3
Cooking Time: 5 Minutes
**Ingredients:**
- ½ cup dragon fruits, peeled and chopped
- ½ cup raspberries (fresh or frozen)
- ½ cup spinach, chopped and washed
- ½ cup mixed greens, washed and chopped
- 1 ripe banana, chopped
- 1-2 dates, pitted
- 1 ½ cups homemade almond milk
- A pinch of cinnamon powder

**Directions:**
1. To your high speed blender, add all the above mentioned items and process on high for 30 seconds. Pour into serving glasses and enjoy immediately.

**Nutrition Info:** (Per Serving): Calories- 320, Fat-7.4 g, Protein- 5 g, Carbohydrates- 62 g

# Pear-simmon Smoothie

Servings: 4
Cooking Time: 5 Minutes
**Ingredients:**
- 4 persimmons, chopped
- 2 small apples, cored and chopped
- 2 small pears, cored and chopped
- 2 handfuls of baby spinach
- 2 cups of mixed greens
- 1 cup filtered water
- 2 teaspoons of freshly squeezed lemon juice
- 4-5 ice cubes

**Directions:**
1. Place all the above ingredients into the blender jar and process until the mixture is thick and creamy.

**Nutrition Info:** (Per Serving): Calories- 239, Fat- 1 g, Protein- 3 g, Carbohydrates- 63 g

# Citrus Coconut Punch

Servings: 2-3
Cooking Time: 5 Minutes
**Ingredients:**
- 1 yellow grapefruit, peeled and deseeded
- 2 mandarins, peeled and deseeded
- 1 large lime, peeled and deseeded
- Freshly squeezed juice of 1 lemon
- 2 cups fresh coconut water
- 1 teaspoon freshly grated ginger
- 4-5 ice cubes

**Directions:**
1. Load all the ingredients into your blender and whizz until smooth.

**Nutrition Info:** (Per Serving): Calories- 211, Fat- 0.6 g, Protein- 4.2 g, Carbohydrates- 53 g

# Nutty Apple Smoothie

Servings: 2
Cooking Time: 2 Minutes
**Ingredients:**
- 2 apple, cored and chopped
- 2/3 cup plain low fat yogurt
- ¼ cup toasted peanuts
- 3 teaspoons raw organic honey
- 1 teaspoon almond butter
- 3-4 ice cubes

**Directions:**
1. Pour all the ingredients into your blender and process until smooth.

**Nutrition Info:** (Per Serving): Calories- 291, Fat- 11g, Protein- 8.3 g, Carbohydrates- 48 g

# Red Healing Potion

Servings: 3
Cooking Time: 5 Minutes
**Ingredients:**
- 2 cups fresh coconut water
- 1 ½ cup pomegranate seeds

- 1 ¼ cup of red grapes, deseeded
- 1 cup whole strawberries ( fresh or frozen)
- 2 tablespoons freshly squeezed lemon juice
- 4-5 ice cubes

**Directions:**
1. Place everything in your blender jar and whizz until smooth and frothy.

**Nutrition Info:** (Per Serving): Calories- 182, Fat-1.2 g, Protein- 4.3 g, Carbohydrates- 44 g

## Cinnaberry Green Smoothie

Servings: 3
Cooking Time: 5 Minutes
**Ingredients:**
- 2 cups unsweetened almond milk
- A handful of baby spinach, washed
- ½ cup mixed greens
- 2 small ripe bananas, sliced (fresh or frozen)
- ½ cup whole raspberries (fresh or frozen)
- 5 teaspoons cacao powder
- 1/3 teaspoon cinnamon powder
- 3-4 ice cubes

**Directions:**
1. To your high speed bender, add all the ingredients and process until smooth.

**Nutrition Info:** (Per Serving): Calories- 375, Fat- 15 g, Protein- 19 g, Carbohydrates- 55 g

## Finana Smoothie

Servings: 2
Cooking Time: 5 Minutes
**Ingredients:**
- 1 banana, chopped (fresh or frozen)
- 2 figs, chopped
- A handful of mixed greens, washed
- ½ cup filtered water
- 1 teaspoon raw organic honey
- 2-3 ice cubes

**Directions:**
1. Load your blender with all the ingredients and puree until smoothie is thick and creamy.

**Nutrition Info:** (Per Serving): Calories- 330, Fat- 1.7 g, Protein- 5.5 g, Carbohydrates- 87 g

## Cherry- Date Plum Smoothie

Servings: 2
Cooking Time: 5 Minutes
**Ingredients:**
- ½ cup cherries, pitted
- 1 zucchini, deseeded and chopped
- 1 plum, pitted and chopped
- 1 teaspoon flax seed powder
- 1-2 dates, pitted
- 1 cup filtered water
- 1 teaspoon freshly squeezed lemon juice
- 3-4 ice

**Directions:**

1. Whizz all the ingredients in the blender until smooth and serve.
**Nutrition Info:** (Per Serving): Calories- 100, Fat- 0.5 g, Protein- 1.8 g, Carbohydrates- 25 g

## Chia Mango-nut Smoothie

Servings: 2
Cooking Time: 5 Minutes
**Ingredients:**
- 1 cup fresh coconut milk
- 1 cup mango, chopped
- 1 tablespoons Chia seeds
- 2 teaspoons freshly squeezed lemon juice
- 2 teaspoons freshly squeezed lime juice
- 2 teaspoons raw organic honey
- 6-7 ice cubes

**Directions:**
1. Dump all the ingredients into the blender and whip it up until the smoothie is thick and creamy.
**Nutrition Info:** (Per Serving): Calories- 211 g, Fat- 11 g, Protein-1.4 g, Carbohydrates-35 g

## Rasp-ricot Smoothie

Servings: 2-3
Cooking Time: 5 Minutes
**Ingredients:**
- 1 ½ cups whole raspberries (fresh or frozen)
- 1 cup low fat plain yogurt
- 2 apricots, pitted and chopped
- 3 teaspoons flax seed powder
- 3 tablespoon raw organic honey
- 4 teaspoons freshly squeezed lemon juice
- 4-5 ice cubes

**Directions:**
1. Place all the above ingredients into the blender jar and process until the mixture is thick and creamy.
**Nutrition Info:** (Per Serving): Calories-289, Fat- 3.5 g. Protein- 12.5 g, Carbohydrates-60 g

## Peachyfig Green Smoothie

Servings: 1 Large
Cooking Time: 2 Minutes
**Ingredients:**
- 1 peach, pitted
- 2 large figs, chopped
- A handful of mixed greens
- ½ cup filtered water
- 2 teaspoon freshly squeezed lemon juice
- 3-4 ice cubes

**Directions:**
1. Place all the ingredients into the blender, secure the lid and whizz on medium high for 30 seconds or until done. Serve immediately.
**Nutrition Info:** (Per Serving): Calories-195, Fat- 1.3 g, Protein- 4.5 g, Carbohydrates- 50 g

## Yogi- Banana Agave Smoothie

Servings: 2-3
Cooking Time: 5 Minutes
**Ingredients:**
- 2 cups plain fat free yogurt
- 2 ripe bananas, chopped
- 3 teaspoon light colored agave nectar
- 2/3 cup blue berries (fresh or frozen)
- 3-4 ice cubes

**Directions:**
1. Pour all the ingredients into your blender and process until smooth.

**Nutrition Info:** (Per Serving): Calories- 275, Fat- 0.6 g, Protein- 11. 5 g. Carbohydrates-c66 g


## Apple Blackberry Wonder

Servings: 2
Cooking Time: 2 Minutes
**Ingredients:**
- 1 cup blackberries (fresh or frozen)
- ½ cup fat free plain yogurt
- 1 tablespoon raw organic honey
- ½ cup freshly prepared apple juice
- ½ banana, sliced
- 2 teaspoon freshly squeezed lemon juice
- 3-4 ice cubes

**Directions:**
1. Add all the above listed items into the blender and blend until well combined.

**Nutrition Info:** (Per Serving): Calories- 260, Fat- 0.9 g, Protein- 5.5 g, Carbohydrates- 64 g


## Date "n" Banana Smoothie

Servings: 2 Small
Cooking Time: X
**Ingredients:**
- 1 large banana, chopped (fresh or frozen)
- 2/3 cup low fat plain yogurt
- 5 medjool dates, pitted
- 1/3 teaspoon nutmeg powder
- 1 teaspoon Chia seeds, soaked
- ½ cup ice cubes

**Directions:**
1. Pour all the ingredients into your blender and process until smooth.

**Nutrition Info:** (Per Serving): Calories- 290, Fat- 1.6 g, Protein- 5.2 g, Carbohydrates- 70 g

# LOW FAT SMOOTHIES

## Banana- Cantaloupe Wonder

Servings: 4
Cooking Time: 5 Minutes
**Ingredients:**
- 2 small banana, chopped
- 4 cups ripe cantaloupe, peeled and chopped
- 1 cup plain non gat yogurt
- 1 teaspoon vanilla extract
- Pinch of cinnamon powder
- ½ cup freshly squeezed orange juice
- 1 teaspoon raw organic honey
- 3-4 ice cubes

**Directions:**
1. Place all the ingredients into your blender and run it on medium high speed for 1-2 minutes or until done.

**Nutrition Info:** (Per Serving): Calories- 360, Fat- 3 g, Protein- 15 g, Carbohydrates- 75 g

## A Batch Of Slimming Berries

Servings: 2
Cooking Time: 5 Minutes
**Ingredients:**
- 1 tablespoon chia seeds
- ¾ cup plain low-fat Greek yogurt
- 1 cup kale
- 1 cup frozen mango
- 1 cup frozen mixed berries
- 1 cup unsweetened vanilla almond milk

**Directions:**
1. Add all the ingredients except vegetables/fruits first
2. Blend until smooth
3. Add the vegetable/fruits
4. Blend until smooth
5. Add a few ice cubes and serve the smoothie
6. Enjoy!

**Nutrition Info:** Calories: 200; Fat: 5g; Carbohydrates: 30g; Protein: 8g

## Berry-chard Smoothie

Servings: 3
Cooking Time: 2 Minutes
**Ingredients:**
- 2 cups rainbow chard, chopped
- 1 large pomegranate, peeled and seeded
- 1 cup mixed berries (fresh or frozen)
- 1 cup fresh, coconut milk
- 3-4 ice cubes

**Directions:**
1. Whizz all the ingredients until well combined and serve.

**Nutrition Info:** (Per Serving): Calories- 80, Fat- 1.5 g, Protein- 2.5 g, Carbohydrates- 41 g

## Cauliflower Cold Glass

Servings: 2
Cooking Time: 5 Minutes
**Ingredients:**
- ½ cup frozen cauliflower, riced
- ½ cup frozen strawberries
- ½ cup frozen blueberries
- ¾ cup plain low-fat Greek yogurt
- 1 fresh banana
- 1 cup unsweetened vanilla almond milk

**Directions:**
1. Add all the ingredients except vegetables/fruits first
2. Blend until smooth
3. Add the vegetable/fruits
4. Blend until smooth
5. Add a few ice cubes and serve the smoothie
6. Enjoy!

**Nutrition Info:** Calories: 204; Fat: 5g; Carbohydrates: 33g; Protein: 8g

## Mango-berry Smoothie

Servings: 3
Cooking Time: 5 Minutes
**Ingredients:**
- ½ cup low fat plain buttermilk
- 1 cup low pat plain yogurt
- ½ lb whole strawberries
- 1 cup mango, peeled and chopped
- 1 small banana, chopped (frozen)
- 1 teaspoon raw organic honey (optional)
- 3-4 ice cubes

**Directions:**
1. Add everything to your blender and pulse it on high for 20 seconds and your smoothie is ready. Enjoy!

**Nutrition Info:** (Per Serving): Calories- 180, Fat- 15 g, Protein-5.5 g, Carbohydrates- 36.5 g

## The Pinky Swear

Servings: 2
Cooking Time: 5 Minutes
**Ingredients:**
- 1 pack (3.5 ounces) frozen dragon fruit
- ¾ cup low-fat Greek yogurt
- 1 cup frozen pineapple
- 1 cup unsweetened coconut milk

**Directions:**
1. Add all the ingredients except vegetables/fruits first
2. Blend until smooth
3. Add the vegetable/fruits
4. Blend until smooth
5. Add a few ice cubes and serve the smoothie
6. Enjoy!

**Nutrition Info:** Calories: 200; Fat: 3g; Carbohydrates: 36g; Protein: 6g

## Berry Nectarine Smoothie

Servings: 2-3

Cooking Time: 2 Minutes
**Ingredients:**
- 2 nectarines, pitted and chopped
- ½ cup whole blueberries (fresh or frozen)
- ½ cup low fat plain yogurt
- ½ teaspoon vanilla extract
- 1 small banana, chopped (fresh or frozen)
- 2-3 ice cubes

**Directions:**
1. To you blender, add the above ingredient and pulse until smooth.

**Nutrition Info:** (Per Serving): Calories- 171, Fat-10 g, Protein- 4.4 g, Carbohydrates- 36 g

## Apple, Dried Figs And Lemon Smoothie

Servings: 2
Cooking Time: 5 Minutes
**Ingredients:**
- 2 medium apples
- ¼ lemon
- A pinch of Himalayan pink salt
- 1 fig, dried

**Directions:**
1. Wash the apples, remove the pit and then roughly chop them
2. Chop the dried fig
3. Toss the chopped apples and figs into your blender
4. Add lemon juice and stir
5. Add a pinch of Himalayan pink salt
6. Serve chilled and enjoy!

**Nutrition Info:** Calories: 120; Fat: 2g; Carbohydrates: 25g; Protein: 5g

## Melon Kiwi Green Melody

Servings: 3
Cooking Time: 2 Minutes
**Ingredients:**
- ½ ripe avocado, peeled and pitted
- ½ ripe banana, sliced
- 1 cup honey dew melon, peeled and chopped
- ½ cup baby spinach, chopped
- ½ cup kale stems removed and chopped
- ½ kiwi, peeled and chopped
- 1/3 cup unsweetened almond milk
- 3-4 ice cubes

**Directions:**
1. Add all the ingredients in the same order as listed above and blend until smooth and thick.

**Nutrition Info:** (Per Serving): Calories- 165, Fat- 7.8 g, Protein- 4.2 g, Carbohydrates- 20 g

## Chai Coconut Shake

Servings: 1
Cooking Time: 10 Minutes
**Ingredients:**
- ¼ cup shredded coconut, unsweetened
- 1 cup coconut milk, unsweetened
- 1 tablespoon pure vanilla extract
- 2 tablespoons almond butter
- 1 teaspoon ginger, grounded

- 1 teaspoon cinnamon, grounded
- 1 tablespoon flaxseed, grounded
- 5 ice cubes
- Pinch of allspice

**Directions:**
1. Add listed ingredients to a blender
2. Blend until you have a smooth and creamy texture
3. Serve chilled and enjoy!

**Nutrition Info:** Calories: 233; Fat: 20g; Carbohydrates: 5g; Protein: 4g

## Berry Banana Blend

Servings: 2
Cooking Time: 2 Minutes
**Ingredients:**
- 1 ripe banana, sliced
- 1 cup whole strawberries (fresh or frozen)
- ½ cup whole blueberries (fresh or frozen)
- ½ cup whole raspberries (fresh or frozen)
- ¾ cup low fat plain yogurt
- 1 teaspoon Chia seeds

**Directions:**
1. Combine all the ingredients in a blender jar and run it for 1 minute or until smooth and creamy.

**Nutrition Info:** (Per Serving): Calories- 225, Fat- 20 g, Protein- 6.2 g, Carbohydrates- 46 g

## Green Tea Berry Classic Smoothie

Servings: 1
Cooking Time: 5 Minutes
**Ingredients:**
- ¼ cups concentrated green tea (1 tea bag+ ¼ cup water)
- ½ cup plain low fat yogurt
- ¼ teaspoon vanilla extract
- 1 ½ teaspoon raw organic honey
- ¼ cup mixed berries
- Pinch of cinnamon powder
- Pinch of nutmeg powder
- 3-4 ice cubes

**Directions:**
1. Combine all the ingredients in a blender jar and run it for 1 minute or until smooth and creamy.

**Nutrition Info:** (Per Serving): Calories- 265, Fat- 4.5 g, Protein- 10 g, Carbohydrates- 50 g

## Papaya, Lemon And Cayenne Pepper Smoothie

Servings: 2
Cooking Time: 5 Minutes
**Ingredients:**
- 2 cups papaya
- ½ teaspoon cayenne pepper
- 3 tablespoons lemon juice

**Directions:**
1. Add all the listed ingredients to a blender
2. Blend until you have a smooth and creamy texture
3. Serve chilled and enjoy!

**Nutrition Info:** Calories: 121; Fat: 6g; Carbohydrates: 20g; Protein: 4g

# Ginger Cantaloupe Detox Smoothie

Servings: 2
Cooking Time: 10 Minutes
**Ingredients:**
- 1 cantaloupe, sliced
- ½ inch ginger, peeled
- 1 tablespoon flaxseed
- 1 pear, chopped
- 1 cup of water
- 1 cup ice

**Directions:**
1. Add all the listed ingredients to a blender except the ginger
2. Blend until smooth
3. Then add ginger and blend again
4. Serve chilled and enjoy!

**Nutrition Info:** Calories: 85; Fat: 2g; Carbohydrates: 19g; Protein: 2g

# Super Veggie Smoothie

Servings: 3- 4
Cooking Time: 5 Minutes
**Ingredients:**
- 1 large carrot, peeled and chopped
- ½ cup broccoli florets
- 1 large apple, cored and chopped
- 2 handfuls of baby spinach, washed and chopped
- 2 large oranges, peeled and seeded
- 1 tablespoons freshly squeezed lemon juice
- ½ cup filtered water

**Directions:**
1. Load your blender jar with the above listed items and process until smooth.

**Nutrition Info:** (Per Serving): Calories- 326, Fat- 1.1 g, Protein- 7.5 g, Carbohydrates- 80 g

# Simple Cherry Berry Wonder

Servings: 3
Cooking Time: 5 Minutes
**Ingredients:**
- ¾ cup whole strawberries (fresh or frozen)
- A handful of blueberries (fresh or frozen)
- ½ cup raspberries (fresh or frozen)
- ½ cup pitted berries (fresh or frozen)
- ½ cup freshly prepared pomegranate juice
- 2 teaspoons freshly squeezed lemon juice
- 3-4 ice cubes

**Directions:**
1. Add all the ingredients in the same order as listed above and blend until smooth and thick

**Nutrition Info:** (Per Serving): Calories-105, Fat- 0.2 g, Protein- 19 g, Carbohydrates- 27 g

# ANTI-AGEING SMOOTHIES

## The Anti-aging Superfood Glass

Servings: 1
Cooking Time: 10 Minutes
**Ingredients:**
- Water as needed
- ½ cup unsweetened nut milk
- 1-2 scoops vanilla Whey Protein
- 1 tablespoon unrefined coconut oil
- 1 tablespoon chia seeds
- 1 tablespoon almond butter
- ¼ cup frozen blueberries
- ½ stick frozen acai puree

**Directions:**
1. Add all the listed ingredients to a blender
2. Blend until you have a smooth and creamy texture
3. Serve chilled and enjoy!

**Nutrition Info:** Calories: 162; Fat: 14g; Carbohydrates: 10g; Protein: 3g

## The Anti-aging Avocado

Servings: 2
Cooking Time: 5 Minutes
**Ingredients:**
- 1 cup ice
- 1 teaspoon vanilla extract
- 1 teaspoon grapeseed oil
- ½ cup avocado, chopped
- ½ cup of frozen strawberries
- ½ cup frozen peaches, chopped
- ½ cup plain Greek yogurt
- ¼ cup 100% pomegranate juice

**Directions:**
1. Add all the ingredients except vegetables/fruits first
2. Blend until smooth
3. Add the vegetable/fruits
4. Blend until smooth
5. Add a few ice cubes and serve the smoothie
6. Enjoy!

**Nutrition Info:** Calories: 447; Fat: 23g; Carbohydrates: 39g; Protein: 22g

## 4 Superfood Spice Smoothie

Servings: 2
Cooking Time: 5 Minutes
**Ingredients:**
- 1 cup unsweetened almond milk
- 1 small banana, chopped (fresh or frozen)
- ¼ cup Goji berries
- 1 teaspoon cacao powder
- 1 teaspoon maca rot powder
- 1 teaspoon hemp seed powder
- 1 teaspoon Chia seeds, soaked

- ¼ teaspoon cinnamon powder
- ½ teaspoon raw organic honey
- 2-3 ice cubes

**Directions:**
1. Add all the ingredients into the blender and process until smooth and thick.

**Nutrition Info:** (Per Serving): Calories- 321, Fat- 15 g, Protein- 13 g, Carbohydrates- 42 g

## Hazelnut And Banana Crunch

Servings: 1 Large
Cooking Time: 2 Minutes
**Ingredients:**
- ¾ cup unsweetened almond milk
- 1 large banana, sliced (fresh or frozen)
- ¼ cup hazelnuts, chopped
- ¼ teaspoon nutmeg powder
- 1 teaspoon raw, organic honey
- 1-2 ice cubes

**Directions:**
1. Add everything to the blender and pulse until smooth. Serve chilled!

**Nutrition Info:** (Per Serving): Calories- 221, Fat- 9.5 g, Protein- 7.8 g, Carbohydrates- 25 g

## A Tropical Glass Of Chia

Servings: 1
Cooking Time: 10 Minutes
**Ingredients:**
- 1 cup coconut water
- 1 tablespoon chia seeds
- 1 cup pineapple, sliced
- ½ cup mango, sliced

**Directions:**
1. Add all the listed ingredients to a blender
2. Blend until you have a smooth and creamy texture
3. Serve chilled and enjoy!

**Nutrition Info:** Calories: 90; Fat: 5g; Carbohydrates: 11g; Protein: 4g

## Powerful Kale And Carrot Glass

Servings: 1
Cooking Time: 10 Minutes
**Ingredients:**
- 1 cup of coconut water
- Lemon juice, 1 lemon
- 1 green apple, core removed and chopped
- 1 carrot, chopped
- 1 cup kale

**Directions:**
1. Add all the listed ingredients to a blender
2. Blend until you have a smooth and creamy texture
3. Serve chilled and enjoy!

**Nutrition Info:** Calories: 116; Fat: 5g; Carbohydrates: 14g; Protein: 6g

## Coconut Mulberry Banana Smoothie

Servings: 3
Cooking Time: 5 Minutes
**Ingredients:**
- 1 cup mulberries (fresh or frozen)
- 2 cups fresh coconut water
- 1/3 cup cranberries
- 1 large banana, chopped (fresh or frozen)
- 1 apple, cored and chopped
- 1 tablespoon hemp seeds
- 1 tablespoon flax seeds
- Freshly squeezed juice of ½ lime
- ½ cup ice cubes

**Directions:**
1. To your high speed blender, add all the items listed above and blitz until everything is well combined.

**Nutrition Info:** (Per Serving): Calories- 322, Fat- 15 g, Protein- 10 g, Carbohydrates- 70 g

## Simple Anti-aging Cacao Dream

Servings: 1
Cooking Time: 10 Minutes
**Ingredients:**
- 1 cup unsweetened almond milk
- 1 tablespoon cacao powder
- 6 strawberries
- 1 banana

**Directions:**
1. Add all the listed ingredients to a blender
2. Blend until you have a smooth and creamy texture
3. Serve chilled and enjoy!

**Nutrition Info:** Calories: 220; Fat: 9g; Carbohydrates: 20g; Protein: 6g

## Lychee- Cucumber Cooler

Servings: 3-4
Cooking Time: 5 Minutes
**Ingredients:**
- 1 ½ cup fresh coconut water
- 1 ½ cup red grapes
- 4-5 lychees, peeled and pitted
- 1 large cucumber, chopped
- 1 handful of spinach
- ½ cup of broccoli florets
- ½ cup chard or kale
- 1 tablespoon lemon juice
- 5-6 cubes of ice

**Directions:**
1. Place all the ingredients into your blender and run in high for 30 seconds or until smooth and frothy. Pour into glasses and serve immediately.

**Nutrition Info:** (Per Serving): Calories 272, - Fat- 1.6 g, Protein- 7 g, Carbohydrates- 70 g

## Super Duper Berry Smoothie

Servings: 2

Cooking Time: 5 Minutes
**Ingredients:**
- ½ cup unsweetened almond milk
- ½ cup frozen blueberries
- ½ cup whole strawberries (fresh or frozen)
- ¼ cup blackberries (fresh or frozen)
- ½ cup red cherries, pitted (fresh or frozen)
- 1 tablespoon cacao powder
- ½ cup romaine lettuce
- 1 teaspoon Chia seeds, soaked
- 1 teaspoon Spirulina powder
- 1 tablespoon hemp powder
- 2-3 ice cubes

**Directions:**
1. To make this smoothie, add all the ingredients into the blender and blitz for 45 seconds on medium high speed.
2. Pour into servings glasses and enjoy!

**Nutrition Info:** (Per Serving): Calories- 345, Fat- 20 g, Protein- 18 g, Carbohydrates- 75 g

## Green Tea-cacao Berry Smoothie

Servings: 2
Cooking Time: 10 Minutes
**Ingredients:**
- 1 cup unsweetened almond or soy milk
- ½ cup strawberries (fresh or frozen)
- ½ cup blueberries ( fresh or frozen)
- ½ cup raspberries (fresh or frozen)
- 1/3 cup freshly brewed green tea
- 1 tablespoon cacao powder
- 3-4 ice cubes

**Directions:**
1. To make the green tea, first takes a sauce pan, bring the water to a boil and take it off the heat.
2. Next add the green tea bag and allow it to steep it for 5 minutes.
3. Allow the tea to cool down to room temperature.
4. Then discard the tea bag.
5. Pour all the ingredients including the tea into the blender jar and run it on medium high for 30 seconds or until smooth.

**Nutrition Info:** (Per Serving): Calories-121, Fat- 2.4 g, Protein- 3.6 g, Carbohydrates- 21 g

## Spiced Blackberry Smoothie

Servings: 2-3
Cooking Time: 5 Minutes
**Ingredients:**
- 1 cup fresh coconut water
- 1 cup whole blackberries (fresh or frozen)
- 1 cup beetroot (peeled and boiled)
- 1 pear, cored and chopped
- ½ cup kale , stems removed and chopped
- 1 tablespoon hemp seed powder
- ¼ teaspoon cinnamon powder
- ¼ teaspoon nutmeg powder
- ½ teaspoon freshly grated ginger

- 1 teaspoon freshly squeezed lemon juice
- 4-5 ice cubes (optional)

**Directions:**

1. Place all the above listed items into the blender and run it on high for 30 seconds until everything is well blended.

**Nutrition Info:** (Per Serving): Calories- 240, Fat-6 g, Protein- 5.1 g, Carbohydrates- 38 g

## Ultimate Orange Potion

Servings: 2
Cooking Time: 5 Minutes
**Ingredients:**

- 1 large carrot, peeled and chopped
- 1 oranges, peeled and deseeded
- ½ cup mango, chopped
- 1-2 celery stalks, chopped
- 1 teaspoon freshly squeezed lemon juice
- ¾ cup filtered water
- 2-3 ice cubes

**Directions:**

1. Combine all the ingredients in a blender and process until smooth.

**Nutrition Info:** (Per Serving): Calories- 113, Fat- 1.1 g, Protein- 3.2 g, Carbohydrates- 26 g

## A Honeydew And Cucumber Medley

Servings: 2
Cooking Time: 5 Minutes
**Ingredients:**

- 1 cup ice
- 1 Medjool date, pitted
- 1 tablespoon ground flaxseed
- 1 tablespoon coconut flour
- ½ lime, juiced
- 1 tablespoon fresh mint, chopped
- 1 cup honeydew
- 1 cup cucumber, chopped
- ¾ cup Greek yogurt

**Directions:**

1. Add all the ingredients except vegetables/fruits first
2. Blend until smooth
3. Add the vegetable/fruits
4. Blend until smooth
5. Add a few ice cubes and serve the smoothie
6. Enjoy!

**Nutrition Info:** Calories: 334; Fat: 7g; Carbohydrates: 50g; Protein: 20g

## Date And Walnut Wonder

Servings: 1 Large
Cooking Time: 2 Minutes
**Ingredients:**

- 8-10 medjool dates, pitted
- 1/3 cup walnuts, halved
- 1 cup unsweetened almond milk

- 3 teaspoons cacao powder
- ½ teaspoon vanilla extract
- ¼ teaspoon cinnamon powder
- A handful of ice cubes

**Directions:**

1. Add everything into the blender jar, secure the lid and process until there are no lumps. Pour into glasses and serve.

**Nutrition Info:** (Per Serving): Calories- 230, Fat- 8.2 g, Protein- 7.9 g, Carbohydrates- 40 g

## Maca – Mango Delight

Servings: 2

Cooking Time: 5 Minutes

**Ingredients:**

- 1 cup fresh coconut water
- 1 cup freshly prepared carrot juice or 1 ½ cup chopped carrot
- 1 large mango, peeled and chopped
- ½ teaspoon maca root powder
- ½ teaspoon cinnamon powder
- 1 teaspoon freshly squeezed lemon juice
- 3-4 ice cubes

**Directions:**

1. Into the blender jar, add all of the ingredients mentioned above and whizz until smooth.

**Nutrition Info:** (Per Serving): Calories- 220, Fat-0 g, Protein- 3 g, Carbohydrates- 10 g

# DIGESTION SUPPORT SMOOTHIES

## Chia-berry Belly Blaster

Servings: 2
Cooking Time: 5 Minutes
**Ingredients:**
- 1 cup berries, frozen
- 1 cup plain Greek yogurt, unsweetened
- 1 tablespoon chia seeds, ground
- 1 tablespoon vanilla extract
- ½ cup ice

**Directions:**
1. Add all the listed ingredients to a blender
2. Blend until you have a smooth and creamy texture
3. Serve chilled and enjoy!

**Nutrition Info:** Calories: 148; Fat: 5g; Carbohydrates: 26g; Protein: 4g

## Tomato- Melon Refreshing Smoothie

Servings: 2
Cooking Time: 2 Minutes
**Ingredients:**
- 1 large tomato, chopped
- 1 ¼ cup watermelon, chopped
- ½ small carrot, peeled and chopped
- 1 teaspoon hemp seeds
- ¾ cup filtered water
- 1 teaspoon freshly squeezed lemon juice
- 3-4 ice cubes

**Directions:**
1. Pour the above listed items into the high speed blender jar and pulse on high for 30 seconds. Pour the smoothie into serving glasses and consume immediately.

**Nutrition Info:** (Per Serving): Calories- 75, Fat- 1.6 g, Protein- 2.9 g, Carbohydrates-16 g

## Blueberry Chia Smoothie

Servings: 2
Cooking Time: 10 Minutes
**Ingredients:**
- 2 cups blueberries, frozen
- 1 cup coconut cream
- 4 tablespoons coconut oil
- 4 tablespoons swerve sweetener
- 4 tablespoons chia seeds, ground
- 2 cups full-fat Greek yogurt
- 2 cups almond milk, unsweetened

**Directions:**
1. Add all the listed ingredients to a blender
2. Blend until you have a smooth and creamy texture
3. Serve chilled and enjoy!

**Nutrition Info:** Calories: 351; Fat: 36g; Carbohydrates: 12.8g; Protein: 12.9g

# Spin-apple Pear Smoothie

Servings: 2-3
Cooking Time: 5 Minutes
**Ingredients:**
- 1 large banana, chipped
- 1 large apple, cored and chopped
- 1 pear, cored and chopped
- 2 cups baby spinach, washed and chopped
- 1 teaspoon raw organic honey (optional)
- 1 cup filtered water
- 2-4 cubes of ice
- A pinch of Celtic salt

**Directions:**
1. Combine everything in the blender jar and pulse until smooth and frothy.

**Nutrition Info:** (Per Serving): Calories- 73, Fat- 3 g, Protein- 4.2 g, Carbohydrates- 19.5 g

# Banana Oatmeal Detox Smoothie

Servings: 2
Cooking Time: 10 Minutes
**Ingredients:**
- 3 tablespoons collard greens
- 3 tablespoons oats
- 1 banana, peeled
- 1 apple, chopped
- 1 teaspoon cinnamon
- 1 cup ice
- 1 cup of water

**Directions:**
1. Add all the listed ingredients to a blender
2. Blend until you have a smooth and creamy texture
3. Serve chilled and enjoy!

**Nutrition Info:** Calories: 162; Fat: 1g; Carbohydrates: 41g; Protein: 3g

# Ginger- Ban-illa Smoothie

Servings: 2
Cooking Time: 2 Minutes
**Ingredients:**
- 1 cup pineapple, chopped (fresh or frozen)
- 1 whole banana, chopped (fresh or frozen)
- 1 cup plain yogurt
- ½ cup filtered water
- ¼ teaspoon vanilla extract
- ½ teaspoon freshly grated ginger
- 3-4 ice cubes

**Directions:**
1. Load your blender with all the above ingredients, secure the lid firmly and whizz it on high for 30 seconds or until well combined.

**Nutrition Info:** (Per Serving): Calories- 200, Fat- 2.3 g, Protein- 8.4 g, Carbohydrates- 37.1 g

# Hemp-melon Refresher

Servings: 1-2
Cooking Time: 2 Minutes

**Ingredients:**
- 1 ½ cup melon, chopped
- 1 large banana, chopped
- 1 teaspoon freshly grated ginger
- 2 teaspoons hemp seed powder
- ¾ cup filtered water
- 2-4 cubes of ice
- 1 inch of cinnamon powder

**Directions:**
1. Place all the items listed above into the blender jar and process until the smoothie is thick and creamy.

**Nutrition Info:** (Per Serving): Calories- 120, Fat- 2 g, Protein- 3.1 g, Carbohydrates- 27 g

## The Pumpkin Eye

Servings: 2
Cooking Time: 5 Minutes

**Ingredients:**
- Dash of ground cinnamon
- 1 tablespoon hemp seeds
- ½ cup unsweetened hemp milk
- ¾ cup Siggi's whole milk vanilla yogurt
- 1 fresh banana
- 1 cup kale
- 1 cup pure canned pumpkin

**Directions:**
1. Add all the ingredients except vegetables/fruits first
2. Blend until smooth
3. Add the vegetable/fruits
4. Blend until smooth
5. Add a few ice cubes and serve the smoothie
6. Enjoy!

**Nutrition Info:** Calories: 216; Fat: 3g; Carbohydrates: 48g; Protein: 3g

## Raspberry Flaxseed Smoothie

Servings: 1 Large
Cooking Time: 2 Minutes

**Ingredients:**
- ½ cup unsweetened almond milk
- ½ cup plain yogurt
- 1 cup raspberries (fresh or frozen)
- 1 large banana, chopped
- 1 tablespoon flaxseeds
- 1 teaspoon freshly squeezed lemon juice
- 2-3 ice cubes

**Directions:**
1. Place all the ingredients into the blender and puree it on high for 3 seconds until smooth and thick.

**Nutrition Info:** (Per Serving): Calories- 160, Fat- 2.2 g, Protein- 7.4 g, Carbohydrates- 30 g

## Vanilla-oats Smoothie

Servings: 2
Cooking Time: 2 Minutes

**Ingredients:**
- 1 large banana, chopped
- ½ cup organic coconut water
- 1 cup plain yogurt

- 4 teaspoons of rolled oats
- ½ teaspoon raw, organic honey
- ½ teaspoon vanilla extract

**Directions:**
1. Combine everything in the blender jar and pulse until creamy.

**Nutrition Info:** (Per Serving): Calories- 220, Fat- 2.5 g, Protein- 10 g, Carbohydrates- 33.5 g

## Matcha Melon Smoothie

Servings: 2
Cooking Time: 5 Minutes
**Ingredients:**
- 1 ½ cups watermelon chopped
- 1 cup unsweetened almond milk
- 1 large bananas, chopped
- 1 ½ teaspoon matcha powder
- 1 teaspoon Chia seeds, soaked
- 1 teaspoon raw, organic honey

**Directions:**
1. Load your high speed blender with everything and process it until thick and creamy. Pour into serving glasses and enjoy.

**Nutrition Info:** (Per Serving): Calories- 273, Fat- 6 g, Protein- 10 g, Carbohydrates- 65 g

## Papaya- Mint Chiller

Servings: 2
Cooking Time: 2 Minutes
**Ingredients:**
- 1 ½ cups papaya, chopped (frozen)
- ½ cup plain yogurt
- 1 tablespoon regularly grated ginger
- 1 tablespoon of freshly squeezed lemon juice
- 1 teaspoon raw, organic honey or liquid Stevia
- 5-7 mint leaves
- A handful of ice cubes

**Directions:**
1. To your blender jar, add the ingredients one by one and process till you get a thick, creamy consistency.

**Nutrition Info:** (Per Serving): Calories- 177, Fat- 1.2 g, Protein-8.2 g, Carbohydrates- 41 g

## Sapodilla, Chia And Almond Milk Smoothie

Servings: 2
Cooking Time: 5 Minutes
**Ingredients:**
- 4 medium sapodillas
- 2/3 cup almond milk
- 3 tablespoons chia seeds
- 1 tablespoon flakes

**Directions:**
1. Wash the sapodillas, peel them and then roughly chop them
2. Toss the chopped sapodillas into your blender
3. Then add almond milk
4. Add all the listed ingredients to a blender
5. Blend well and add almond on top
6. Serve and enjoy!

**Nutrition Info:** Calories: 113; Fat: 1g; Carbohydrates: 21g; Protein: 5g

## Grape And Nectarine Blende

Servings: 1
Cooking Time: 5 Minutes
**Ingredients:**
- 1 cup red or green grapes, seedless
- 1 large nectarine, peeled and chopped
- 1 cup plain yogurt
- 1 teaspoon freshly squeezed lemon juice
- 1 teaspoon raw organic honey
- ¼ teaspoon cinnamon powder
- 1/3 cup filtered water

**Directions:**
1. To your high speed blender jar, add the ingredients and puree it until creamy and thick.

**Nutrition Info:** (Per Serving): Calories- 201, Fat- 2.2 g, Protein- 8.9 g, Carbohydrates- 32 g


## A Minty Drink

Servings: 2
Cooking Time: 5 Minutes
**Ingredients:**
- 1 tablespoon hemp seeds
- Fresh mint leaves
- ¾ cup plain coconut yogurt
- 1 cup frozen mango
- 1 cup frozen strawberries
- 1 cup unsweetened vanilla almond milk

**Directions:**
1. Add all the ingredients except vegetables/fruits first
2. Blend until smooth
3. Add the vegetable/fruits
4. Blend until smooth
5. Add a few ice cubes and serve the smoothie
6. Enjoy!

**Nutrition Info:** Calories: 391; Fat: 10g; Carbohydrates: 44g; Protein: 5g


## The Nutty Macadamia Delight

Servings: 1
Cooking Time: 10 Minutes
**Ingredients:**
- Oz Macadamia nuts
- 1 cup spinach
- 1 tablespoon chia seeds
- 1 packet stevia, if you want
- 2/3 cup water
- ¼ cup heavy cream

**Directions:**
1. Add all the listed ingredients into your blender
2. Blend until smooth
3. Serve chilled and enjoy!

**Nutrition Info:** Calories: 485; Fat: 48g; Carbohydrates: 13g; Protein: 7g

# ANTI-INFLAMMATORY SMOOTHIES

## Nutty Banana & Ginger Smoothie

Servings: 4
Cooking Time: 10 Minutes
**Ingredients:**

- 1 frozen banana, peeled and sliced
- ¼-inch fresh turmeric root, grates
- ½-inch fresh ginger root, peeled and chopped
- 1 cup pecans, chopped
- 1 cup walnuts, chopped
- 1 tablespoon flax seeds
- 1 tablespoon chia seeds
- 1 tablespoon fresh maca powder
- ½ teaspoon ground cinnamon
- 1½ cups unsweetened almond milk

**Directions:**

1. In a high speed blender, add all ingredients and pulse till smooth.
2. Transfer into 4 glasses and serve immediately.

## Chia And Cherry Smoothie

Servings: 1
Cooking Time: 5 Minutes
**Ingredients:**

- A handful of fresh cherries
- ½ cup of pineapple, cubed
- A couple of beetroot pieces
- 1 tablespoon of Chia seeds
- 2-3 ice cubes (optional)
- 8 ounces of coconut water
- 1 teaspoon of coconut oil

**Directions:**

1. Wash the cherries, pineapple and beetroot before chipping them and place in a blender.
2. Add the remaining ingredients to the jar and run it on high for 1 minute until smooth.
3. Serve chilled.

**Nutrition Info:** (Per Serving): Calories- 250, Fat-4.5 g, Protein- 6 g, Carbohydrates-51 g

## Apple, Strawberry & Beet Smoothie

Servings: 4
Cooking Time: 10 Minutes
**Ingredients:**

- 2 cups frozen strawberries, hulled and sliced
- 1 beet, peeled and chopped
- 1 cup apple, peeled, cored and sliced
- 3 Medjool dates, pitted and chopped
- ¼ cup extra virgin coconut oil
- ½ cup unsweetened almond milk

**Directions:**

1. In a high speed blender, add all ingredients and pulse till smooth.
2. Transfer into a glass and serve immediately.

**Nutrition Info:** (Per Serving):Calories: 223.4, Fat: 14.6g, Carbohydrates: 22.3g, Fiber: 3.9g, Protein: 1.5g, Sodium: 49.7mg

## Tangy Ginger & Radish Smoothie

Servings: 2
Cooking Time: 10 Minutes
**Ingredients:**
- 1 orange, peeled, seeded and sliced
- 1 radish, trimmed and chopped
- 1 tablespoon fresh ginger, peeled and chopped
- 5-10 fresh mint leaves
- 1 tablespoon ground chia seeds
- 1 teaspoon organic honey
- 1 cup spring water
- ½ cup fresh orange juice
- 1 tablespoon fresh lemon juice
- Ice, as required

**Directions:**
1. In a high speed blender, add all ingredients and pulse till smooth.
2. Transfer into 2 glasses and serve immediately.


## Spinach & Berries Smoothie

Servings: 1
Cooking Time: 10 Minutes
**Ingredients:**
- 1 cup mixed frozen berries (blueberries, strawberries, cranberries)
- 2 cups fresh spinach
- 1 cup celery stalk, chopped
- 2-inch pieces fresh ginger, peeled and chopped
- 3 tablespoons hemp protein powder
- ½ cup filtered water

**Directions:**
1. In a high speed blender, add all ingredients and pulse till smooth.
2. Transfer into a glass and serve immediately.


## Pineapple & Coconut Smoothie

Servings: 1
Cooking Time: 10 Minutes
**Ingredients:**
- 1 cup fresh pineapple, diced
- 1 tablespoon coconut, shredded
- ½ lime, peeled and seeded
- 1 tablespoon chia seeds
- 1 teaspoon ground turmeric
- Pinch of freshly ground black pepper
- ½ cup coconut water

**Directions:**
1. In a high speed blender, add all ingredients and pulse till smooth.
2. Transfer into a glass and serve immediately.

## Guava Berry Smoothie

Servings: 2
Cooking Time: 5 Minutes
**Ingredients:**
- ½ guava, chopped
- 1 cup strawberries (fresh or frozen)
- 2 bananas (fresh or frozen)
- 4 cups spinach, washed
- 6 ounces of filtered water

**Directions:**
1. Load the blender with all the ingredients and whip it up for 1 minute until smooth.
2. Pour in a tall glass and enjoy!

**Nutrition Info:** (Per Serving): Calories-339, Fat 2g, Protein- 9.1 g, Carbohydrates-81 g

## Cherry & Blueberry Smoothie

Servings: 1
Cooking Time: 10 Minutes
**Ingredients:**
- 2 cups escarole
- ½ cup frozen blueberries
- ½ cup frozen cherries
- ¼ teaspoon ground cinnamon
- ¼ teaspoon ground turmeric
- 1 scoop of chocolate protein powder
- 1 cup filtered water
- 5 ice cubes, crushed

**Directions:**
1. In a high speed blender, add all ingredients and pulse till smooth.
2. Transfer into a glass and serve immediately.

## Kale And Apple Smoothie

Servings: 2
Cooking Time: 5 Minutes
**Ingredients:**
- 2 cups of fresh kale, washed and chopped
- 1 apple, cored and chopped
- 1 orange, peeled and deseeded
- 1 cup of filtered water

**Directions:**
1. Place all the ingredients into a blender and blend until smooth.

**Nutrition Info:** (Per Serving): Calories-125, Fat-2 g, Protein- 8 g, Carbohydrates- 61 g

## Pineapple & Almond Smoothie

Servings: 3
Cooking Time: 10 Minutes
**Ingredients:**
- 1 cup fresh pineapple, peeled and chopped
- ¼ cup blanched almonds
- ½ cup fresh pineapple juice
- ½ teaspoon pure maple syrup
- ½ cup fresh pineapple juice

- ¼ cup rice milk
- ½ cup ice cubes, crushed

**Directions:**
1. In a high speed blender, add all ingredients and pulse till smooth.
2. Transfer into a glass and serve immediately.

**Nutrition Info:** (Per Serving):Calories: 96.7, Fat: 5.2g, Sat Fat: 0.5g, Carbohydrates: 11.6g, Fiber: 1.3g, Protein: 2.5g

## Sweet And Spicy Fruit Punch

Servings: 1
Cooking Time: 10 Minutes
**Ingredients:**
- 1 cup freshly brewed green tea (room temperature or chilled)
- ½ cup papaya, chopped (fresh or frozen)
- ½ cup avocado, chopped
- ½ cup of blueberries (fresh or frozen)
- 1 tablespoon of Chia seeds
- A handful of baby spinach
- A pinch of cayenne pepper
- ½ teaspoon of freshly grated turmeric
- ½ teaspoon of freshly grated ginger
- ½ teaspoon of cinnamon powder
- 1 teaspoon of raw, organic honey
- 1 teaspoon of coconut oil
- A pinch of sea salt

**Directions:**
1. Brew a fresh cup of green tea and allow it to cool.
2. If you prefer chilled smoothie, refrigerate this tea for 1 hour.
3. Next, add all the dry ingredients into the blender and process until well combined.
4. Then, pour in the wet ingredients and blend it for 30 seconds more till the desired consistency is got.
5. Serve immediately.

**Nutrition Info:** (Per Serving): Calories 264, Fat 13 g, Protein- 4.1 g, Carbohydrates- 41 g

## Spiced Peach Smoothie

Servings: 2
Cooking Time: 10 Minutes
**Ingredients:**
- ½ of frozen banana, peeled and chopped
- 1 cup frozen peaches, pitted and chopped
- ½ teaspoon ground ginger
- ½ teaspoon chia seeds
- 1 teaspoon ground turmeric
- 1 teaspoon ground cinnamon
- 1 teaspoon raw honey
- 10-ounce unsweetened almond milk

**Directions:**
1. In a high speed blender, add all ingredients and pulse till smooth.
2. Transfer into a glass and serve immediately.

## Fruit & Veggie Smoothie

Servings: 2

Cooking Time: 15 Minutes
**Ingredients:**
- ¾ cups pineapple, chopped
- ½ cup cucumber, peeled and chopped
- ½ of pear, peeled, cored and chopped
- 1 small avocado, peeled, pitted and chopped
- ½ tablespoon fresh dill
- 1 cup fresh spinach, chopped
- 1 celery stalk, chopped
- ¼ teaspoon ground turmeric
- 1 piece fresh ginger, peeled
- 1 tablespoon fresh lime juice
- 2 cups water

**Directions:**
1. In a high speed blender, add all ingredients and pulse till smooth.
2. Transfer into 2 glasses and serve immediately.


## Cherry & Kale Smoothie

Servings: 1
Cooking Time: 10 Minutes
**Ingredients:**
- 2 ripe bananas, peeled and sliced
- 1 cup fresh cherries, pitted
- 1 cup fresh kale, trimmed
- 1 teaspoon fresh ginger, peeled and chopped
- 1 tablespoon chia seeds, soaked for 15 minutes
- ½ teaspoon ground turmeric
- ¼ teaspoon ground cinnamon
- 1 cup coconut water

**Directions:**
1. In a high speed blender, add all ingredients and pulse till smooth.
2. Transfer into a glass and serve immediately.


## Turmeric-mango Smoothie

Servings: 2
Cooking Time: 5 Minutes
**Ingredients:**
- 2 cups unsweetened almond milk
- 1 banana (fresh or frozen)
- 1 cup papaya, chopped (fresh or frozen)
- 1 cup mango, chopped
- 1 teaspoon freshly grated turmeric
- Pinch of black pepper
- ½ teaspoon finely grated ginger
- 1 tablespoon raw organic honey
- ½ teaspoon vanilla extract

**Directions:**
1. For this recipe, you need to prepare a turmeric milk concoction before you make the smoothie.
2. Heat a sauce pan on medium high and boil the almond milk, along with the turmeric, black pepper, ginger and honey.
3. Let it simmer for 5 minutes on low.
4. Allow this mixture to cool completely.

5. Once it has cooled, load your blender with this concoction, and all the remaining ingredients and process it until smooth.
**Nutrition Info:** (Per Serving): Calories-262, Fats-10 g, Proteins- 5.8 g, Carbohydrates-40.6 g

## Spiced Banana Smoothie

Servings: 1
Cooking Time: 10 Minutes
**Ingredients:**
- 2 bananas, peeled and sliced
- 2 teaspoons ground ginger
- ½ teaspoon ground turmeric
- ½ teaspoon organic vanilla extract
- 1 tablespoon honey
- 1 cup coconut milk
- 6-8 ice cubes, crushed

**Directions:**
1. In a high speed blender, add all ingredients and pulse till smooth.
2. Transfer into a glass and serve immediately.

# MUSCLE, BONE AND JOINT SMOOTHIES

## Coconut-blueberry Smoothie

Servings: 3
Cooking Time: 5 Minutes
**Ingredients:**
- 1 cup fresh coconut water
- 1 cup blueberries
- 1 large banana, sliced (fresh or frozen)
- 1 cup baby spinach, washed and chopped
- ½ cup fresh kale, stems removed and chopped
- ½ cup dandelion greens chopped
- 1 teaspoon freshly squeezed lemon juice

**Directions:**
1. Place all the ingredients into the blender and blitz until smooth.

**Nutrition Info:** (Per Serving): Calories- 250, Fat- 1.1 g, Protein- 4 g, Carbohydrates- 60 g

## Ginger- Papaya Smoothie

Servings: 2
Cooking Time: 5 Minutes
**Ingredients:**
- 1 cup plain yogurt
- 1 ¼ cup papaya, chopped
- 1 tablespoon raw organic honey
- ¼ teaspoon freshly grated ginger
- 1 teaspoon freshly squeezed lemon juice
- 4-5 ice cubes

**Directions:**
1. Add all the ingredients into the blender, secure the lid and pulse into smooth.

**Nutrition Info:** (Per Serving): Calories- 140, Fat- 3.4 g, Protein- 6.1 g, Carbohydrates- 25 g

## Pineapple Sage Smoothie

Servings: 2
Cooking Time: 5 Minutes
**Ingredients:**
- 1 cup pineapple, peeled and chopped
- 1 pear, core and chopped
- 2-3 sage leaves
- 1 teaspoon Chia seeds, soaked
- 1 teaspoon hemp seed powder
- 1 teaspoon freshly squeezed lemon juice
- ¾ cup water
- 2-3 ice cubes

**Directions:**
1. Add all the ingredients into the blender and run it on high for 30 seconds or until well combined.

**Nutrition Info:** (Per Serving): Calories- 250, Fat- 1.1 g, Protein- 5 g , Carbohydrates- 87 g

## Orange Sunrise Smoothie

Servings: 3
Cooking Time: 5 Minutes
**Ingredients:**

- ¾ cup coconut water
- 2 large carrots, peeled and chopped
- 2 cups pineapple, chopped
- 1 cup freshly squeezed orange juice
- 1 cup lightly packed iceberg lettuce
- 2-3 celery stalks chopped
- 3 teaspoons Chia seeds, soaked
- ½ teaspoon freshly grated ginger

**Directions:**
1. To the blender, add all the ingredients and pulse until smooth.

**Nutrition Info:** (Per Serving): Calories- 345, Fat- 3 g, Protein- 7.5 g, Carbohydrates- 55g

## Fruit "n" Nut Smoothie

Servings: 2
Cooking Time: 5 Minutes
**Ingredients:**
- 1 cup freshly brewed green tea
- 1 cup red cherries, pitted
- 1 cup whole strawberries (fresh or frozen)
- ½ kale, stems removed
- ¼ cup walnuts, halved
- ½ teaspoon freshly grated ginger
- 1 teaspoon wheat grass powder
- 1 teaspoon hemp powder

**Directions:**
1. Load all the ingredients in a high speed blender and process until it is smooth and thick.

**Nutrition Info:** (Per Serving): Calories- 255, Fat- 11 g, Protein- 8.9 g, Carbohydrates- 38 g

## Maca –banana Smoothie

Servings: 2-3
Cooking Time: 5 Minutes
**Ingredients:**
- 1 cup fresh coconut water
- 1 tablespoon almond butter
- 1 ½ medium banana, chopped (fresh or frozen)
- ½ tablespoon maca powder
- ½ cup fresh baby spinach, washed and chopped
- 1 teaspoon Chia seeds
- A pinch of cinnamon powder
- 2-3 ice cubes

**Directions:**
1. Load the blender with all the ingredients and process on medium speed for 30 second or until smoothie is thick and creamy.

**Nutrition Info:** (Per Serving): Calories- 430, Fat- 19.8 g, Protein- 12 g, Carbohydrates- 58 g

## Ginger- Parsely Grape Smoothie

Servings: 1
Cooking Time: 2 Minutes
**Ingredients:**
- 1 ½ cup red grapes, seedless
- ½ cup parsley, washed and chopped

- 2 tablespoons avocado flesh
- ¼ cup freshly squeezed lemon juice
- 1 teaspoon freshly grated ginger
- 3 drops of liquid Stevia or ½ teaspoon raw organic honey
- 4-5 mint leaves
- A handful of ice cubes

**Directions:**
1. Add all the ingredients into the blender and blitz until smooth.

**Nutrition Info:** (Per Serving): Calories- 230, Fat- 5.4 g, Protein- 3.9 g, Carbohydrates- 55 g

## Spinach And Kiwi Smoothie

Servings: 2-3
Cooking Time: 2 Minutes
**Ingredients:**
- 1 cup fresh coconut milk
- 1 ½ cup fresh baby spinach
- ½ cup arugula, chopped
- 1 cup kiwi, peeled and chopped
- 1 small banana, chopped
- 1 teaspoon freshly squeezed lemon juice

**Directions:**
1. Add all the ingredients to a high speed blender and pulse until smooth. Pour into glasses and serve.

**Nutrition Info:** (Per Serving): Calories- 130, Fat- 2.1 g, Protein- 2 g, Carbohydrates- 29 g

## Berry-cantaloupe Smoothie

Servings: 3
Cooking Time: 5 Minutes
**Ingredients:**
- ½ cup whole strawberries (fresh or frozen)
- 1 cup mango, chopped
- 1 cups cantaloupe, chopped
- ½ cup fresh kale, stems removed
- 1 celery stalks, chopped
- 1 chard leaves, chopped
- A small handful of parsley
- ¼ cup baby spinach
- ½ cup filtered water

**Directions:**
1. Pour all the ingredients into a high speed blender and run in on high for 2 seconds or until the desired consistency is got.

**Nutrition Info:** (Per Serving): Calories- 375, Fat- 1.9 g, Protein- 6.8 g, Carbohydrates- 95 g

## Apple –kiwi Blush

Servings: 2
Cooking Time: 5 Minutes
**Ingredients:**
- 1 cup unsweetened almond milk
- 1 large apple, cored and chopped
- 2 kiwi fruits, peeled and chopped
- 1 cup cucumber, chopped
- 2-3 collard green leaves, stems removed and chopped
- 3 teaspoons Chia seeds, soaked
- 2-3 ice cubes (optional)

**Directions:**

1. Place all the ingredients in a high speed bender and blitz on medium speed for 30 seconds or until smooth.
**Nutrition Info:** (Per Serving): Calories- 340, Fat- 0.5 g, Protein- 11 g, Carbohydrates- 60 g

## Cucumber- Pear Healer

Servings: 2
Cooking Time: 2 Minutes
**Ingredients:**
- 1 cup unsweetened almond milk
- 2 cups cucumber, chopped
- 2 large pears, cored and chopped
- 8-9 fresh mint leaves
- 1 teaspoon freshly squeezed lemon juice
- 1 teaspoon raw organic honey
- 3-4 ice cubes

**Directions:**
1. Just add all the ingredients into the blender and pulse until smooth.
**Nutrition Info:** (Per Serving): Calories- 285, Fat- 4.8 g, Protein- 5 g, Carbohydrates- 65 g

## Cucumber- Pineapple

Servings: 3
Cooking Time: 5 Minutes
**Ingredients:**
- 1 ¼ cups fresh coconut water
- 1 cup cucumber, chopped
- ½ cup pineapple, chopped
- 1 small avocado, peeled and chopped
- 1/3 cup fresh kale, stems removed
- 1/3 cup baby spinach
- ½ teaspoon freshly grated ginger

**Directions:**
1. Combine all the ingredients in a high speed blender and pulse until smooth.
**Nutrition Info:** (Per Serving): Calories- 260, Fat- 15 g, Protein- 7 g, Carbohydrates- 22 g

## Ginger Lime Smoothie

Servings: 3
Cooking Time: 5 Minutes
**Ingredients:**
- 1 cup fresh coconut water
- Freshly squeezed juice of 1 lime
- 1 cup pineapple, chopped
- 1 cup kale, stems removed and chopped
- ½ banana, chopped (fresh or frozen)
- ½ cup arugula
- 1-2 celery stalks, chopped
- 6-7 mint leaves
- ½ teaspoon freshly grated ginger
- 1 ½ teaspoon Chia seeds, soaked
- 2-4 ice cubes

**Directions:**
1. Place all the above listed ingredients into your blender and blend until smooth. Enjoy immediately.
**Nutrition Info:** (Per Serving): Calories- 345, Fat- 4 g, Protein- 8.5 g, Carbohydrates- 75 g

# Banana- Guava Smoothie

Servings: 3-4
Cooking Time: 5 Minutes
**Ingredients:**
- 2 large bananas, chopped (fresh or frozen)
- ½ cup strawberries (fresh or frozen)
- ½ cup raspberries (fresh or frozen)
- 1 cup guava, peeled, deseeded and chopped
- 1 cup baby spinach
- ½ cup dandelion greens
- ½ cup romaine lettuce
- ½ cup water
- 1-2 ice cubes

**Directions:**
1. Pour all the ingredients into a high speed blender and process it on high for 20 seconds or until smooth and creamy.

**Nutrition Info:** (Per Serving): Calories- 325, Fat- 1.9 g, Protein- 10 g, Carbohydrates- 82 g

# Kiwi Quick Smoothie

Servings: 2
Cooking Time: 2 Minutes
**Ingredients:**
- ½ cup unsweetened almond milk
- ½ cup plain yoghurt
- ¼ cup fresh coconut milk
- ½ cup whole strawberries (fresh or frozen)
- 1 kiwi, peeled and chopped
- 1 teaspoon raw, organic honey
- ½ teaspoon Chia seeds

**Directions:**
1. Combine all the ingredients in a high speed blender and process until smooth.

**Nutrition Info:** (Per Serving): Calories- 260, Fat- 9 g, Protein- 13 g, Carbohydrates- 37 g

# Orange Gold Smoothie

Servings: 2
Cooking Time: 5 Minutes
**Ingredients:**
- ½ cup fresh coconut milk
- ½ cup mango, chopped
- ½ cup pineapple, chopped
- ½ cup peaches, pitted
- ½ teaspoon freshly grated lemon zest
- ¼ teaspoon cinnamon powder
- ¼ teaspoon nutmeg powder
- ½ teaspoon cayenne pepper
- A pinch of Celtic salt
- ¾ cup filtered water
- A handful of ice cubes

**Directions:**
1. Place all the ingredients into the blender and whizz until thick and smooth.

**Nutrition Info:** (Per Serving): Calories- 171, Fat- 4.4 g, Protein- 2.9 g, Carbohydrates- 35 g

# SUPERFOOD SMOOTHIES

## Chia Flax Berry Green Smoothie

Servings: 3
Cooking Time: 5 Minutes
**Ingredients:**
- 1 cup unsweetened almond milk
- 2 teaspoons almond butter
- 1 cup frozen mixed berries
- 1 ripe banana, chopped
- 1 cup fresh spinach, chopped
- 2 teaspoons flaxseed powder
- 2 teaspoons Chia seeds oaked
- 1 teaspoon raw organic honey
- 4-5 ice cubes

**Directions:**
1. Whizz all the ingredients until well combined and serve.

**Nutrition Info:** (Per Serving): Calories- 360, Fat- 1.3 g, Protein- 11 g, Carbohydrates- 45 g

## Hemp, Date And Chia Smoothie

Servings: 2
Cooking Time: 2 Minutes
**Ingredients:**
- 1 cup unsweetened almond milk
- ¼ teaspoon vanilla extract
- 1 dates, pitted
- 1 tablespoon hemp seeds
- ½ ripe banana, chopped
- 1 teaspoon Chia seeds, soaked
- A large handful of chopped kale
- 4-5 ice cubes

**Directions:**
1. Place all the ingredients into your blender and run it on medium high speed for 1-2 minutes or until done.

**Nutrition Info:** (Per Serving): Calories- 218, Fat- 11 g, Protein- 8 g, Carbohydrates- 31 g

## Oat And Walnut Berry Blast

Servings: 2
Cooking Time: 2 Minutes
**Ingredients:**
- ¼ cup rolled oats
- ¼ cup walnuts, chopped
- 1 cup whole blueberries (fresh or frozen)
- 2 oranges, peeled and seeded
- 1 teaspoon cinnamon powder
- 1 cup filtered water
- 3-4 ice cubes

**Directions:**
1. Whizz all the ingredients until well combined and serve.

**Nutrition Info:** (Per Serving): Calories- 218, Fat- 8 g, Protein- 6 g, Carbohydrates- 35 g

# Aloe Vera Smoothie

Servings: 3
Cooking Time: 5 Minutes
**Ingredients:**
- ½ cup pure aloe Vera gel
- ½ ripe avocado, peeled and pitted
- Freshly squeezed juice of ½ lime
- 1 ½ teaspoon pure coconut oil
- 1 cup mixed greens, washed and chopped
- 1 kiwi, peeled and chopped
- 1 teaspoon flax seed powder
- 1 teaspoon Chia seeds
- A pinch of Celtic salt
- 1 teaspoon raw organic honey
- 1 cup filtered water
- 4-5 ice cubes
- 1 teaspoon freshly squeezed lemon juice

**Directions:**
1. Add all the ingredients in the same order as listed above and blend until smooth and thick

**Nutrition Info:** (Per Serving): Calories- 360, Fat- 31 g, Protein- 3.2 g, Carbohydrates- 35 g

# Raspberry Peach Delight

Servings: 3
Cooking Time: 5 Minutes
**Ingredients:**
- 1 cup whole raspberries (fresh or frozen)
- 1 ½ cups peaches, pitted (fresh or frozen)
- 1 cup unsweetened, organic coconut milk
- ¼ teaspoon vanilla extract
- 2 teaspoons Chia seeds
- 2 teaspoons freshly squeezed lemon juice
- 2 teaspoons raw organic honey
- 1 cups filtered water
- 4-5 ice cubes

**Directions:**
1. To you blender, add the above ingredient and pulse until smooth.

**Nutrition Info:** (Per Serving): Calories- 161, Fat- 4.9 g, Protein- 3 g, Carbohydrates- 30 g

# Berry Melon Green Smoothie

Servings: 3
Cooking Time: 5 Minutes
**Ingredients:**
- ¾ cup watermelon, chopped
- ½ cup whole strawberries (fresh or frozen)
- 1 ½ cup fresh baby spinach, washed and chopped
- 1 ripe banana, chopped
- 1 cup fresh coconut water
- Freshly squeezed juice of ½ lime
- 1 ½ teaspoon flaxseed powder
- 3-4 ice cubes

**Directions:**
1. Add all the ingredients in the same order as listed above and blend until smooth and thick

**Nutrition Info:** (Per Serving): Calories- 121, Fat- 1.5 g, Protein- 3 g, Carbohydrates- 25 g

## Blue And Green Wonder

Servings: 3
Cooking Time: 5 Minutes
**Ingredients:**
- 1 cup unsweetened almond milk
- 1 cup whole blueberries (fresh or frozen)
- 1 ripe banana, chopped
- 1 cup baby spinach, washed and chopped
- 1 cup fresh kale, stems removed and chopped
- 2 teaspoons flax seeds
- 4-5 ice cubes

**Directions:**
1. Add all the ingredients in the same order as listed above and blend until smooth and thick

**Nutrition Info:** (Per Serving): Calories- 122, Fat- 2 g, Protein- 3 g, Carbohydrates- 25 g

## Raspberry Carrot Smoothie

Servings: 2
Cooking Time: 5 Minutes
**Ingredients:**
- 1 large carrot, peeled and chopped
- 1 cup whole raspberries (fresh or frozen)
- ½ cup low fat plain yogurt
- 4 teaspoons Goji berries
- 1 tablespoon Chia seeds
- 1 tablespoon flaxseed powder
- 1 teaspoon raw organic honey
- 4-5 ice cubes

**Directions:**
1. To your high speed blender, add all the ingredients and pulse until smooth.

**Nutrition Info:** (Per Serving): Calories- 335, Fat- 12 g, Protein- 13.5 g, Carbohydrates- 45 g

## Green Tea Superfood Smooothie

Servings: 4
Cooking Time: 5 Minutes
**Ingredients:**
- ½ cup freshly prepared pomegranate juice
- 1 cup freshly brewed green tea (unsweetened and chilled)
- ½ cup plain low fat Greek yogurt
- 1 cup mixed berries (fresh or frozen)
- 1 ripe banana, chopped (fresh or frozen)
- 1 large handful baby spinach, washed and chopped
- 1 teaspoon freshly grated ginger
- 1 teaspoon flaxseed powder
- 3-4 ice cubes

**Directions:**
1. To make this smoothie, add all the ingredients into your high speed blender and puree until smooth.

**Nutrition Info:** (Per Serving): Calories-130, Fat- 1 g, Protein- 6.9 g, Carbohydrates- 27 g

# Nutty Mango Green Blend

Servings: 2
Cooking Time: 5 Minutes
**Ingredients:**
- 1 cup fresh mango, chopped (fresh or frozen)
- 1 cup fresh baby spinach, washed and chopped
- ½ cup low fat plain yogurt
- 1 teaspoon pistachios
- 1 teaspoon peanuts
- 1 teaspoon pecan nuts
- ½ teaspoon liquid Stevia
- 2 teaspoons freshly squeezed lemon juice
- 5 ice cubes

**Directions:**
1. To you blender, add the above ingredient and pulse until smooth.
**Nutrition Info:** (Per Serving): Calories-300, Fat- 6.8 g, Protein- 12 g, Carbohydrates- 45 g


# Super Tropi-kale Wonder

Servings: 4
Cooking Time: 5 Minutes
**Ingredients:**
- 1 cup pineapple, chopped
- 1 cup mango, peeled and hopped
- 2 cups mixed greens, washed and chopped
- 1 ripe banana, chopped
- 1 teaspoon Spirulina powder
- ½ teaspoon bee pollen
- 3 teaspoons Brazil nuts
- 2 teaspoons flax seeds
- 1 ½ teaspoon pure coconut oil
- 1 ¼ cup filtered water
- 3-4 ice cubes

**Directions:**
1. Add all the ingredients in the same order as listed above and blend until smooth and thick.
**Nutrition Info:** (Per Serving): Calories- 300, Fat-11 g, Protein-7.4 g, Carbohydrates-45 g


# Choco- Berry Delight

Servings: 4
Cooking Time: 5 Minutes
**Ingredients:**
- ½ cup whole blueberries (fresh or frozen)
- ½ cup cherries, pitted
- 1 ripe banana, chopped
- 1 cup unsweetened almond milk
- 2 cups mixed greens, washed and chopped
- 1 cup baby spinach, washed and chopped
- 2 stalks celery, copped
- 2 teaspoons raw cacao powder
- 1teapoon Chia seeds
- 3-4 ice cubes

**Directions:**
1. Place all the ingredients into your blender and run it on medium high speed for 1-2 minutes or until done.

**Nutrition Info:** (Per Serving): Calories- 310, Fat- 7.9 g, Protein- 8 g, Carbohydrates- 59 g

## Carrot Crunch Smoothie

Servings: 2
Cooking Time: 5 Minutes
**Ingredients:**
- 1 grapefruit, peeled and seeded
- 1 cup carrot, peeled and chopped
- 1 cup low fat plain yogurt
- 2 teaspoons raw, organic honey
- 3 teaspoons macadamia nuts, chopped
- 3 teaspoons almonds, chopped
- 5-6 ice cubes

**Directions:**
1. Place all the ingredients into the high speed blender jar and run it on high for 20 seconds until everything is well combined. Pour into serving glass and enjoy!

**Nutrition Info:** (Per Serving): Calories- 310, Fat- 12 g, Protein- 11 g, Carbohydrates- 39 g

## Coconut Blue Wonder

Servings: 2
Cooking Time: 5 Minutes
**Ingredients:**
- 1 cup whole blueberries (fresh or frozen)
- 1 cup organic coconut milk
- ¼ cup plain low fat yogurt
- 1 small handful of baby spinach, chopped
- 1 ½ teaspoon flaxseed powder
- 3-4 ice cubes

**Directions:**
1. Combine all the ingredients in a blender jar and run it for 1 minute or until smooth and creamy.

**Nutrition Info:** (Per Serving): Calories- 240, Fat- 11 g, Protein- 4 g, Carbohydrates- 31 g

## Banana-sunflower Coconut Smoothie

Servings: 2
Cooking Time: 2 Minutes
**Ingredients:**
- 2 ripe bananas, sliced (fresh or frozen)
- 3 teaspoons raw cacao powder
- 2 teaspoons maca powder
- 3 teaspoons coconut cream
- 2 teaspoon sunflower seeds
- 1 cup filtered water
- 1 teaspoon raw organic honey
- 4-5 ice cubes

**Directions:**
1. Place all the ingredients into your blender and run it on medium high speed for 1-2 minutes or until done.

**Nutrition Info:** (Per Serving): Calories- 200, Fat- 6.9 g, Protein- 3.6 g, Carbohydrates- 32 g

# Tea And Grape Smoothie

Servings: 2
Cooking Time: 5 Minutes

**Ingredients:**
- 1 large apple, cored and chopped
- 1 cup red grapes, seedless
- ½ cup freshly brewed green tea (unsweetened and chilled)
- ½ cup plain low fat yogurt
- 1 teaspoons raw organic honey
- 1 teaspoons freshly grated ginger
- 3-4 ice cubes

**Directions:**
1. Load your high speed blender jar with all the ingredients and puree until thick and smooth.

**Nutrition Info:** (Per Serving): Calories- 131, Fat- 1 g, Protein- 5 g, Carbohydrates- 25 g

# GREEN SMOOTHIES

## Tropical Matcha Kale

Servings: 2
Cooking Time: 5 Minutes
**Ingredients:**
- ½ cup ice
- 1 cup kale, chopped
- ½ cup frozen mango died
- 1 teaspoon matcha powder
- ½ cup plain kefir
- ¼ cup cold water

**Directions:**
1. Add all the ingredients except vegetables/fruits first
2. Blend until smooth
3. Add the vegetable/fruits
4. Blend until smooth
5. Add a few ice cubes and serve the smoothie
6. Enjoy!

**Nutrition Info:** Calories: 126; Fat: 2g; Carbohydrates: 23g; Protein: 6g

## Cilantro And Citrus Glass

Servings: 2
Cooking Time: 5 Minutes
**Ingredients:**
- ½ cup ice
- 2 cups arugula
- ½ cup celery, diced
- 1 grapefruit, peeled and segmented
- 1 handful fresh cilantro leaves, chopped
- ½ lemon, juiced
- ½ cup water

**Directions:**
1. Add all the ingredients except vegetables/fruits first
2. Blend until smooth
3. Add the vegetable/fruits
4. Blend until smooth
5. Add a few ice cubes and serve the smoothie
6. Enjoy!

**Nutrition Info:** Calories: 75; Fat: 1g; Carbohydrates: 16g; Protein: 3g

## Glowing Green Smoothie

Servings: 2
Cooking Time: 10 Minutes
**Ingredients:**
- 2 bananas
- 2 kiwis
- 4 celery stalks
- ½ cup pineapple
- 2 cups of water
- 4 cups spinach

**Directions:**

1. Add all the listed ingredients to a blender
2. Blend until you have a smooth and creamy texture
3. Serve chilled and enjoy!
**Nutrition Info:** Calories: 191; Fat: 1.1g; Carbohydrates: 46.5g; Protein: 7.8g

## Lovely Green Gazpacho

Servings: 2
Cooking Time: 5 Minutes
**Ingredients:**
- ½ cup ice
- 1 cup collard greens, chopped
- ¼ cup red bell pepper, diced
- ½ cup frozen broccoli florets
- ½ cup fresh tomatoes, chopped
- 1 garlic clove
- ¼ cup fresh cilantro, chopped
- ½ lemon, juiced
- ½ cup water

**Directions:**
1. Add all the ingredients except vegetables/fruits first
2. Blend until smooth
3. Add the vegetable/fruits
4. Blend until smooth
5. Add a few ice cubes and serve the smoothie
6. Enjoy!
**Nutrition Info:** Calories: 70; Fat: 1g; Carbohydrates: 13g; Protein: 4g

## Berry Spinach Basil Smoothie

Servings: 2
Cooking Time: 5 Minutes
**Ingredients:**
- 1 cup unsweetened almond milk
- 1 small banana, chopped
- ½ cup blueberries (fresh or frozen)
- A small handful of baby spinach
- 6-7 fresh basil leaves
- 2 teaspoons freshly squeezed lemon juice
- 3-4 ice cubes

**Directions:**
1. Add all the ingredients into the high speed blender and whizz until smooth.
**Nutrition Info:** (Per Serving): Calories- 250, Fat- 5.8g, Protein- 5 g ,Carbohydrates- 51 g

## Garden Variety Green And Yogurt Delight

Servings: 1
Cooking Time: 10 Minutes
**Ingredients:**
- 1 cup whole milk yogurt
- 1 tablespoon flaxseed, ground
- 1 cup garden greens
- 1 tablespoon MCT oil
- 1 cup of water

- 1 pack stevia

**Directions:**
1. Add listed ingredients to a blender
2. Blend until you have a smooth and creamy texture
3. Serve chilled and enjoy!

**Nutrition Info:** Calories: 334; Fat: 26g; Carbohydrates: 14g; Protein: 11g

## Mixed Berry Basil Green Smoothie

Servings: 3
Cooking Time: 5 Minutes
**Ingredients:**
- 1 ripe banana, chopped
- 1/3 cup fresh basil, washed
- 1 cup fresh spinach, washed
- ¼ cup blueberries (fresh or frozen)
- ¼ cup raspberries (fresh or frozen)
- ¼ cup strawberries (fresh or frozen)
- ¼ cup blackberries (fresh or frozen)
- 1 teaspoon Chia seeds. Soaked
- ½ teaspoon flax seeds
- 1 teaspoon coconut flakes
- 2 teaspoon coconut oil
- 1 teaspoon raw organic honey
- ¼ teaspoon cinnamon powder
- 1 cup filtered water

**Directions:**
1. Add all the ingredients into the high speed blender and whizz until smooth.

**Nutrition Info:** (Per Serving): Calories- 300, Fat- 15 g, Protein- 3.2 g, Carbohydrates- 45 g

## Lettuce Plum Smoothie

Servings: 3-4
Cooking Time: 5 Minutes
**Ingredients:**
- ¾ cup unsweetened almond milk
- 1 ½ cup escarole or romaine lettuce, washed and chopped
- ½ cup whole cranberries (fresh or frozen)
- 1 cup banana, sliced
- 2 large plums, pitted and chopped
- 1 teaspoon freshly squeezed lemon juice
- ½ teaspoon raw organic homey
- 3-4 ice cubes

**Directions:**
1. Combine all the ingredients in a high speed blender and whirr until thick and smooth.

**Nutrition Info:** (Per Serving): Calories-383, Fat-2.1 g, Protein- 11 g, Carbohydrates- 93 g

## Dandelion Green Berry Smoothie

Servings: 2
Cooking Time: 5 Minutes
**Ingredients:**
- ½ cup dandelion greens, chopped
- ½ small banana, hopped

- A handful of mixed berries
- 1 cup filtered water
- 1 teaspoon coconut oil
- A pinch of cinnamon powder
- 1 teaspoon flax seed powder
- 1 teaspoon cacao powder
- 1 teaspoon raw organic honey
- ½ teaspoon Chia seeds
- ½ teaspoon hemp seeds
- 3-4 ice cubes

**Directions:**
1. Add all the above listed ingredients into your blender, secure the lid and blitz until smooth.

**Nutrition Info:** (Per Serving): Calories- 270, Fat- 16 g, Protein- 3.2 g, Carbohydrates- 35 g

## Berry Spirulina Smoothie

Servings: 2
Cooking Time: 2 Minutes
**Ingredients:**
- ½ cup blueberries (fresh or frozen)
- 1 cup spinach, chopped
- ½ avocado, peeled , pitted and chopped
- 1 tablespoon Spirulina powder
- 1 teaspoon raw cacao powder
- 1 teaspoon flax seed powder
- 1 teaspoon Chia seeds
- 1 teaspoon maca root powder
- 1 teaspoon raw organic honey
- A pinch of cinnamon power
- A pinch of Celtic salt
- ½ cup filtered water
- 3-4 ice cubes

**Directions:**
1. Blend all the ingredients into the blender and enjoy!

**Nutrition Info:** (Per Serving): Calories-260, Fat- 14 g, Protein- 6.8 g, Carbohydrates- 30 g

## Lemon Cilantro Delight

Servings: 2
Cooking Time: 5 Minutes
**Ingredients:**
- ½ cup ice
- 1 cup dandelion greens, chopped
- 2 celery stalks, roughly chopped
- 1 pear, roughly chopped
- 1 tablespoon chia seeds
- ¼ cup fresh cilantro, chopped
- Juice of ½ lemon
- ¼ cup water

**Directions:**
1. Add all the ingredients except vegetables/fruits first
2. Blend until smooth
3. Add the vegetable/fruits
4. Blend until smooth

5. Add a few ice cubes and serve the smoothie
6. Enjoy!
**Nutrition Info:** Calories: 200; Fat: 5g; Carbohydrates: 34g; Protein: 5g

## Orange Grapefruit Green Smoothie

Servings: 3
Cooking Time: 2 Minutes
**Ingredients:**
- 1 large apple, cored and chopped
- 1 pink grapefruits, peeled and deseeded
- 1 large banana, sliced (frozen)
- ½ cup freshly squeezed orange juice
- 2 cups fresh spinach, washed
- ½ teaspoon freshly grated ginger
- ½ teaspoon raw, organic honey
- 3-4 ice cubes

**Directions:**
1. To make this smoothie, place everything into the blender and pulse until smooth. Serve immediately.
**Nutrition Info:** (Per Serving): Calories- 130, Fat- 5 g, Protein- 2 g, Carbohydrates 30 g

## Pineapple And Cucumber Cooler

Servings: 3-4
Cooking Time: 5 Minutes
**Ingredients:**
- 1 green apple, cored and chopped
- 1 cup pineapple, peeled and chopped
- 1 green cucumber, deseeded and chopped
- 5-6 celery stalks, chopped
- A handful of kale leaves, stems removed and chopped
- 1/3 cup fresh parsley
- 1 teaspoon freshly grated ginger
- 1 tablespoon freshly squeezed lemon juice
- 3-4 ice cubes

**Directions:**
1. Add all the ingredients into the blender jar and pulse it on high for 30 seconds or until smooth.
**Nutrition Info:** (Per Serving): Calories-226, Fat- 1.8 g, Protein- 7.8 g, Carbohydrates- 36 g

## Berry Collard Green Smoothie

Servings: 3
Cooking Time: 5 Minutes
**Ingredients:**
- ½ avocado, pitted and chopped
- 1 small banana, chopped
- ½ cup coconut water
- ½ cup collard greens, chopped
- ½ cup pineapple, peel and chopped
- ¾ cup whole blueberries (fresh or frozen)
- 1 teaspoon freshly squeezed lemon juice
- ¼ teaspoon freshly grated ginger
- ½ teaspoon raw, organic honey
- 4-5 ice cubes

**Directions:**
1.  Place all the ingredients in the blender and run it on high for 30 seconds or until the desired consistency is got.
**Nutrition Info:** (Per Serving): Calories- 166, Fat-1.8 g, Protein- 5 g, Carbohydrates- 42 g

## Greenie Genie S Moothie

Servings: 3
Cooking Time: 5 Minutes
**Ingredients:**
*   1 cup unsweetened almond milk
*   1 banana, chopped (fresh or frozen)
*   ½ cup avocado, pitted and chopped
*   1 kiwi fruit, peeled and chopped
*   1 cup baby spinach, chopped
*   1 tablespoons raw organic honey
*   A pinch of cinnamon powder
*   3-4 ice cubes
**Directions:**
1.  Add all the ingredients into the blender and whizz until smooth.
**Nutrition Info:** (Per Serving): Calories- Fat- 4.5 g, Protein- 5 g, Carbohydrates- 17 g

## Citrus Green Smoothie

Servings: 2
Cooking Time: 10 Minutes
**Ingredients:**
*   2 oranges, peeled
*   2 cups almond milk
*   1 cup strawberries
*   2 cups spinach, raw
**Directions:**
1.  Add listed ingredients to a blender
2.  Blend until you have a smooth and creamy texture
3.  Serve chilled and enjoy!
**Nutrition Info:** Calories: 334; Fat: 28.9g; Carbohydrates: 20.8g; Protein: 4.3g

# VEGAN AND VEGETARIAN DIET SMOOTHIES

## Healthy Kiwi Smoothie

Servings: 2
Cooking Time: 20 Min
**Ingredients:**
- 1 celery stalk
- 2 medium granny smith apples, cored
- 1 kiwi fruit, peeled and chopped
- 1/3 cup parsley leaves
- 1 tbsp. grated ginger
- Maple syrup
- 2 tsp lime juice

**Directions:**
1. Add all ingredients in a blender, except lime juice and blend until smooth. Taste and adjust sweetness with maple syrup.
2. Stir in lime juice and serve.

**Nutrition Info:** (Per Serving): Cal 82 Total Fat 1 g, Carbs 20 g, Fiber 0 g, Protein 1 g, Sodium 9 mg Sugars 18 g

## Apple, Carrot, Ginger & Fennel Smoothie

Servings: 2
Cooking Time: 5 Min
**Ingredients:**
- 1 medium apple
- 2 medium carrots
- 2 tablespoons peeled ginger slices
- 1 cup sliced fennel bulb
- 1 tablespoon honey
- 1 cup apple juice
- 1 tablespoons lemon juice
- 1 cup ice cubes

**Directions:**
1. Peel and core apple, cut into slices and place in a blender.
2. Peel carrots, dice and add to blender along with ginger, fennel bulb, honey, apple juice, lemon juice and ice cubes.
3. Pulse for 1 minute until smoothie and serve immediately.

**Nutrition Info:** (Per Serving):144 Cal, 0 g total fat (0 g sat. fat), 0 mg chol., 63 mg sodium, 36 g carb., 5g fiber, 2 g protein.

## Beet And Grapefruit Smoothie

Servings: 1
Cooking Time: 5 Min
**Ingredients:**
- 1/2 Cucumber, peeled and diced
- 1/2 small red beet, peeled and diced
- 1 apple, cored and chopped
- 6 tbsps. Grapefruit juice
- 4 ice cubes

**Directions:**
1. In a high speed blender, add cucumber and blend until it breaks into pieces. Add apple, beet and blend until smooth.

2. Add water if it's too hard to blend. Push the sides and blend again until you reach fine consistency. Add ice, grapefruit juice and blend.
3. Serve right away.
**Nutrition Info:** (Per Serving): Cal 208 Total Fat 1.2 g, Carbs 45.9 g, Fiber 4 g, Protein 6 g, Sodium 33 mg Sugars 25 g

## Raspberry Smoothie

Servings: 2
Cooking Time: 5 Min
**Ingredients:**
- 1 cup water
- 1 cup frozen raspberries
- 1 large sliced frozen bananas
- 2 tbsps. Lime juice
- 1 tsp coconut oil
- 1 tsp agave syrup

**Directions:**
1. In a high-speed blender, add all ingredients and process until smooth.
2. You can add ice if you want or add more frozen bananas. Adjust taste with agave syrup.
**Nutrition Info:** (Per Serving): Cal 480 Total Fat 1 g, Carbs 126 g, Fiber 9 g, Protein 2 g, Sodium 20 mg Sugars 28 g

## Spinach, Grape, & Coconut Smoothie

Servings: 2
Cooking Time: 5 Min
**Ingredients:**
- 2 cups seedless green grapes
- 2 cups baby spinach
- ½ cup reduced fat coconut milk
- 1 cup ice cubes

**Directions:**
1. In a blender, place grapes, spinach and ice, and pour in milk.
2. Pulse for 1 minute until smooth and serve immediately.
**Nutrition Info:** (Per Serving):194 Cal, 2 g total fat (0 g sat. fat), 0 mg chol., 108 mg sodium, 31 g carb., 4g fiber, 0 g protein.

## Chard, Lime & Mint Smoothies

Servings: 2
Cooking Time: 5 Min
**Ingredients:**
- 5 ½ ounces honeydew melon
- 3 ounces kiwifruit
- 2 cups green Swiss chards
- ½ cup soda, lime-flavored
- ¼ cup chopped mint
- 3 tablespoons reduced fat vanilla milk
- ⅛ Teaspoon salt
- 3 tablespoons lime juice
- 1 cup ice cubes

**Directions:**
1. Peel and core melon, cut into cubes and place in a blender.

2. Peel and core kiwifruit and add to melon along with soda, mint and milk.
3. Remove stems of chards, discard, discard leaves into strips and add to blender.
4. Add ice and pulse for 1 minute until smooth. Add more lime juice if smoothie is thick.
5. Serve immediately.
**Nutrition Info:** (Per Serving):67 Cal, 0.7 g total fat (0 g sat. fat), 0 mg chol., 267 mg sodium, 16 g carb., 3g fiber, 2 g protein.

## Mango, Lime & Spinach Smoothie

Servings: 2
Cooking Time: 5 Min
**Ingredients:**
- 1 cup seedless green grapes
- 2 cups baby spinach
- 1 large Mango
- 2 tablespoons lime juice
- 1 cup ice cubes

**Directions:**
1. Peel and core mango, roughly chop flesh and place in a blender.
2. Add grapes, spinach, lime juice, ice and pulse for 1 minute until smooth.
3. Serve immediately.
**Nutrition Info:** (Per Serving):167 Cal, 0 g total fat (0 g sat. fat), 0 mg chol., 67 mg sodium, 64 g carb., 5g fiber, 6 g protein.

## Super Avocado Smoothie

Servings: 2
Cooking Time: 5 Min
**Ingredients:**
- 1 medium avocado
- 1 cup blueberries
- 1 cup frozen strawberries
- ½ cup frozen raspberries
- ¼ cup reduced fat vanilla yogurt
- 1 cup orange juice
- ½ cup filtered water
- 1 tablespoon maple syrup
- 15 mint leaves

**Directions:**
1. Peel and pit avocado and add to a blender.
2. Add blueberries, strawberries, raspberries, yogurt, orange juice, water, maple syrup and mint.
3. Pulse for 1 minute until smooth and serve immediately.
**Nutrition Info:** (Per Serving):156 Cal, 8 g total fat (1 g sat. fat), 0 mg chol., 64 mg sodium, 54 g carb., 8g fiber, 3 g protein.

## Chia, Blueberry & Banana Smoothie

Servings: 2
Cooking Time: 5 Min
**Ingredients:**
- 2 medium fresh bananas
- 1 cup frozen blueberries
- 1 cup fat free milk, unsweetened
- 2 tablespoons Chia Seeds

- 1 cup ice cubes

**Directions:**
1. Peel banana, chop roughly and place in a blender along with blueberries, milk, chia seeds and ice.
2. Pulse 1 minute until smooth and serve immediately.

**Nutrition Info:** (Per Serving):220 Cal, 1.5 g total fat (0.5 g sat. fat), 0 mg chol., 71 mg sodium, 48 g carb., 3.4g fiber, 5.5 g protein.

## Mango Smoothie

Servings: 2
Cooking Time: 5 Min
**Ingredients:**
- 1 1/2 cups orange juice
- 1/2 cup water
- 1/4 cup sliced avocado
- 1/2 tsp lime zest, grated
- 2 cups frozen sweet mango
- 1 tsp maple syrup

**Directions:**
1. Place all the ingredients in a blender. Blend until smooth and fine texture. Add more water if too thick and blend again.
2. To adjust sweetness, add more maple syrup. Enjoy while still cold!

**Nutrition Info:** (Per Serving): Cal 270 Total Fat 1.5 g, Carbs 53 g, Fiber 6 g, Protein 16 g, Sodium 0 mg Sugars 37 g

## Pina Colada Smoothie

Servings: 2
Cooking Time: 5 Min
**Ingredients:**
- 1 cup pineapple chunks
- 1 banana
- 2 teaspoons honey
- 1 cup reduced fat coconut milk, unsweetened
- ½ cup ice cubes
- 2 Pineapple wedges, for garnish

**Directions:**
1. Peel banana, chop roughly and place in a blender along with pineapple, honey, coconut milk and ice cubes.
2. Pulse for 1 minute until smooth and divide smoothie between two serving glasses.
3. Garnish each serving glass with a pineapple wedge and serve immediately.

**Nutrition Info:** (Per Serving):158 Cal, 6.6 g total fat (2 g sat. fat), 0 mg chol., 39 mg sodium, 23 g carb., 2g fiber, 2.7 g protein.

## Avocado And Blueberry Smoothie

Servings: 2
Cooking Time: 10 Min
**Ingredients:**
- 1 cup orange juice
- 1/2 cup mineral water
- 1 haas avocado, seeded and peeled
- 1 cup fresh blueberries
- 1/4 cup vegan yogurt
- 1 tbsp. maple syrup

- 1 cup frozen blueberries
- 1/2 cup frozen raspberries
- 1/4 cup fresh mint leaves
- Pinch of Celtic salt

**Directions:**
1. Throw everything in a high speed blender. Process until smooth.
2. Serve right away.

**Nutrition Info:** (Per Serving): Cal 111 Total Fat 12.3 g, Carbs 39.2 g, Fiber 8.1 g, Protein 11 g, Sodium 206 mg Sugars 29 g

## Chai Tea Smoothie

Servings: 2
Cooking Time: 10 Min
**Ingredients:**
- 1 cup unsweetened almond milk
- 1 cup coconut juice
- 1/4 cup chopped dates, soaked
- 1 tsp vanilla extract
- 1/2 tsp cinnamon powder
- 1/4 tsp ginger powder
- 1/8 tsp nutmeg powder
- 1/8 tsp cardamom powder
- Pinch of cloves powder
- Pinch of Himalayan sea salt
- 2 large frozen bananas, sliced
- 1 cup crushed ice
- 1 tbsp. chia seeds

**Directions:**
1. Add everything in a high-speed blender. Blend until smooth and creamy.
2. Serve right away!

**Nutrition Info:** (Per Serving): Cal 227 Total Fat 1 g, Carbs 52 g, Fiber 6 g, Protein 3 g, Sodium 280 mg Sugars 35 g

## Strawberry Watermelon Smoothie

Servings: 2
Cooking Time: 5 Min
**Ingredients:**
- 1 1/2 cups sliced watermelons, seeds removed
- 1 cup frozen strawberries
- 1/2 frozen ripe banana, sliced
- 1/2 cup unsweetened almond milk
- 1 lime juice
- 1 tbsp. chia seeds

**Directions:**
1. Add all ingredients in a blender. Process until smooth and fine texture. Adjust sweetness with more banana.
2. Top with more chia seeds.

**Nutrition Info:** (Per Serving): Cal 182 Total Fat 6.2 g, Carbs 30 g, Fiber 9 g, Protein 5 g, Sodium 48 mg Sugars 14 g

## Caramel Banana Smoothie

Servings: 2

Cooking Time: 10 Min

**Ingredients:**

- 1 1/2 cups almond milk
- 3 Medjool dates, pitted
- 2 medium frozen bananas, sliced
- 1 scoop of Vegan Vanilla Ice Cream
- 1 tbsp. almond butter

**Directions:**

1. Add everything in a blender and blend until smooth.
2. Garnish with some shaved chocolate on top or serve as is.

**Nutrition Info:** (Per Serving): Cal 140 Total Fat 7 g, Carbs 13 g, Fiber 2 g, Protein 7 g, Sodium 330 mg Sugars 60 g

## Green Smoothie

Servings: 2

Cooking Time: 5 Min

**Ingredients:**

- 2 medium green apples
- Half of a medium avocado
- 1-inch ginger piece
- 1 cup baby spinach
- 1 cup coconut water
- 1 tablespoon flax oil
- 1 cup ice cubes

**Directions:**

1. Peel apple, core, slice and place in a blender. Peel and pit avocado and add to blender.
2. Peel and dice ginger and add to blender along with spinach, coconut water, flax oil and ice cubes.
3. Pulse for 1 minute until smooth and creamy and then serve over ice.

**Nutrition Info:** (Per Serving):156 Cal, 1 g total fat (0.2 g sat. fat), 0 mg chol., 54 mg sodium, 38 g carb., 6.5g fiber, 3.6 g protein.

# BRAIN HEALTH SMOOTHIES

## Cacao-goji Berry Marvel

Servings: 2 Small
Cooking Time: 5 Minutes
**Ingredients:**
- 1 cup unsweetened almond milk
- 1 large banana, chopped (preferably frozen)
- ¼ cup Goji berries
- 3-4 fresh kale leaves, stems removed
- 1 ½ teaspoon cacao powder
- 3 teaspoon almond butter
- ¼ teaspoon cinnamon powder
- 4-6 ice cubes

**Directions:**
1. Load your blender with all the smoothie ingredients and process it on medium speed until the smoothie is ready. Serve immediately.

**Nutrition Info:** (Per Serving): Calories- 345, Fat- 10 g, Protein- 12 g, Carbohydrates- 57 g

## Brewed Green Tea Smoothie

Servings: 4
Cooking Time: 10 Minutes
**Ingredients:**
- 2 large avocados, pitted and peeled
- 4 cups spinach
- ½ cup fresh mint leaves
- 2 cups green tea, brewed and cooled
- 4 stalks celery, chopped
- 2 grapefruits, peeled and frozen
- 4 cups pineapple, chunked and frozen
- ¼ teaspoon ground cayenne pepper

**Directions:**
1. Add all the listed ingredients to a blender
2. Blend until you have a smooth and creamy texture
3. Serve chilled and enjoy!

**Nutrition Info:** Calories: 155; Fat: 0.4g; Carbohydrates: 8g; Protein: 5.6g

## Mango- Chia- Coconut Smoothie

Servings: 3
Cooking Time: 5 Minutes
**Ingredients:**
- 2 cups unsweetened organic coconut milk
- 1 cup mixed berries (fresh or frozen)
- 1 cup mango, chopped (fresh or frozen)
- 1 cup fresh kale, stems removed and chopped
- 1 large banana, chopped (fresh or frozen)
- 2 tablespoons Chia seeds, soaked
- 3 teaspoons of cashew butter
- ¼ cup of filtered water

**Directions:**
1. Add all the ingredients into the blender jar one by one, secure the lid firmly and whizz for 30 seconds or until done.

**Nutrition Info:** (Per Serving): Calories- 170, Fat- 6.8 g, Protein- 5 g, Carbohydrates- 25 g

## Nutty Bean "n"berry Smoothie

Servings: 2-3
Cooking Time: 5 Minutes
**Ingredients:**
- 1 cup blueberries (fresh or frozen)
- 1 cup whole strawberries (fresh or frozen)
- 1 large, raw brazil nut (roughly chopped)
- ½ cup cannellini beans (soaked overnight, drained and rinsed)
- 2 teaspoons sunflower seeds
- 2 teaspoon flax seed powder
- 1 ½ cups of filtered water

**Directions:**
1. Load your high speed blender jar with all the ingredients and puree until thick and smooth.

**Nutrition Info:** (Per Serving): Calories- 163, Fat- 6.4 g, Protein- 6.3 g, Carbohydrates- 23 g

## Cinnammon-apple Green Smoothie

Servings: 2
Cooking Time: 5 Minutes
**Ingredients:**
- ¾ cup unsweetened almond milk
- 1 cup fresh kale, stems removed
- 1 cup baby spinach, washed and chopped
- 1 large apple, peeled, cored and chopped
- 1 large banana, chopped (fresh or frozen)
- 1 teaspoon raw, organic honey
- ½ teaspoon cinnamon powder
- 3-4 ice cubes

**Directions:**
1. To your blender jar, add all the above mentioned ingredients and process until smooth.

**Nutrition Info:** (Per Serving): Calories-243, Fat- 3.2 g, Protein- 4.5 g, Carbohydrates- 47 g

## Chia-hemp Berry Smoothie

Servings: 2
Cooking Time: 5 Minutes
**Ingredients:**
- 1 cup unsweetened almond milk
- 1 cup whole strawberries (fresh or frozen)
- ¼ cup blueberries (fresh or frozen)
- ¼ cup raspberries (fresh or frozen)
- ¼ cup lack berries 9fresh or frozen)
- ¼ cup cranberries 9fresh or frozen)
- 3 tablespoons chopped almonds
- 3 teaspoons almond butter
- 3 teaspoons hemp seeds
- 2 teaspoons Chia seeds, soaked

**Directions:**
1. Place the ingredients into the blender, secure the lid and blend until the smoothie is nice and thick.

**Nutrition Info:** (Per Serving): Calories- 266, Fat- 17.8 g, Protein- 7 g, Carbohydrates- 26.3 g

# Cucumber Kiwi Crush

Servings: 2
Cooking Time: 5 Minutes
**Ingredients:**
- 1 cup green cucumber, roughly chopped
- 1 large kiwi, peeled and chopped
- ½ cp plain low fat yogurt
- ½ cup freshly prepared tangerine juice
- 1 cup fresh baby spinach, washed and chopped
- ½ avocado, peeled and chopped
- 1 teaspoon of freshly squeezed lemon juice
- A small handful of mint leaves
- A handful of ice cubes

**Directions:**
1. Combine all the ingredients in the blender and process until there are no lumps. Serve immediately.

**Nutrition Info:** (Per Serving): Calories-185, Fat- 7.8 g, Protein- 5.2 g, Carbohydrates- 32 g

# Matcha Coconut Smoothie

Servings: 2
Cooking Time: 5 Minutes
**Ingredients:**
- 3 tablespoons white beans
- ½ teaspoon matcha green tea powder
- 1 whole banana, cubed
- 1 cup of frozen mango, chunked
- 2 kale leaves, torn
- 2 tablespoon coconut, shredded
- 1 cup of water

**Directions:**
1. Add all the listed ingredients to a blender
2. Blend on high until you have a smooth and creamy texture
3. Serve chilled and enjoy!

**Nutrition Info:** Calories: 291; Fat: 25g; Carbohydrates: 18g; Protein: 5g

# Muscular Macho Green

Servings: 2
Cooking Time: 5 Minutes
**Ingredients:**
- 2 teaspoons matcha powder
- 1 tablespoon chia seeds
- ¾ cup plain coconut yogurt
- 1 fresh banana
- 1 cup baby spinach
- 1 cup frozen mango
- 1 cup unsweetened coconut milk

**Directions:**
1. Add all the ingredients except vegetables/fruits first
2. Blend until smooth
3. Add the vegetable/fruits
4. Blend until smooth
5. Add a few ice cubes and serve the smoothie
6. Enjoy!

**Nutrition Info:** Calories: 200; Fat: 5g; Carbohydrates: 35g; Protein: 6g

## A Whole Melon Surprise

Servings: 2
Cooking Time: 5 Minutes
**Ingredients:**
- 1 tablespoon chia seeds
- 4 ice cubes
- 1 fresh banana
- 1 cup cantaloupe
- 1 cup honeydew
- 1 cup plain coconut yogurt
- 1 cup unsweetened coconut milk

**Directions:**
1. Add all the ingredients except vegetables/fruits first
2. Blend until smooth
3. Add the vegetable/fruits
4. Blend until smooth
5. Add a few ice cubes and serve the smoothie
6. Enjoy!

**Nutrition Info:** Calories: 134; Fat: 2g; Carbohydrates: 29g; Protein: 3g

## The Wisest Watermelon Glass

Servings: 2
Cooking Time: 5 Minutes
**Ingredients:**
- 1 tablespoon chia seeds
- 1 cup plain coconut yogurt
- 1 cup frozen cauliflower, riced
- 1 cup frozen strawberries
- 1 cup coconut milk, unsweetened
- 1½ cups watermelon, chopped

**Directions:**
1. Add all the ingredients except vegetables/fruits first
2. Blend until smooth
3. Add the vegetable/fruits
4. Blend until smooth
5. Add a few ice cubes and serve the smoothie
6. Enjoy!

**Nutrition Info:** Calories: 130; Fat: 2g; Carbohydrates: 22g; Protein: 8g

## Hale 'n' Kale Banana Smoothie

Servings: 1
Cooking Time: 2 Minutes
**Ingredients:**
- 1 cup fresh kale, chopped (stems removed)
- 1 handful blueberries (fresh or frozen)
- 1 small banana, chopped (fresh or frozen)
- ½ teaspoon Chia seeds
- ½ cup filtered water

**Directions:**

1. Add the kale, berries, banana, Chia seeds and water into your blender jar and process on high for 20 seconds or until smooth and frothy.

**Nutrition Info:** (Per Serving): Calories- 201, Fat- 1.2 g, Protein- 3.9 g, Carbohydrates- 44 g

## Buddha's Banana Berry

Servings: 2
Cooking Time: 5 Minutes
**Ingredients:**
- 1 tablespoon hemp seeds
- ¾ cup plain low-fat Greek yogurt
- 1 fresh banana
- 1 cup baby spinach
- 1 cup frozen raspberries
- 1 cup unsweetened vanilla almond milk

**Directions:**
1. Add all the ingredients except vegetables/fruits first
2. Blend until smooth
3. Add the vegetable/fruits
4. Blend until smooth
5. Add a few ice cubes and serve the smoothie
6. Enjoy!

**Nutrition Info:** Calories: 205; Fat: 1g; Carbohydrates: 51g; Protein: 3g

## Sweet Pea Smoothie

Servings: 2
Cooking Time: 10 Minutes
**Ingredients:**
- 2 cups sweet peas
- 1 cup blueberries
- 1 teaspoon honey
- 2 bananas
- 2 cups almond milk
- 2 tablespoons chia seeds

**Directions:**
1. Add all the listed ingredients to a blender
2. Blend until you have a smooth and creamy texture
3. Serve chilled and enjoy!

**Nutrition Info:** Calories: 202; Fat: 4.1g; Carbohydrates: 38.4g; Protein: 6.8g

## Berry Infusion Smoothie

Servings: 2
Cooking Time: 2 Minutes
**Ingredients:**
- ½ cup freshly prepared pomegranate juice
- ½ large banana, chopped (fresh or frozen)
- ½ cup blueberries (fresh or frozen)
- ½ cup raspberries (fresh or frozen)
- A handful of pineapple chunks
- 2 tablespoons Chia seeds, soaked
- A few ice cubes

**Directions:**

1. Add all the ingredients into your blender jar, secure the lid firmly and whizz for 30 seconds or until the smoothie is thick and creamy.
**Nutrition Info:** (Per Serving): Calories- 378, Fat- 4.5 g, Protein- 25 g, Carbohydrates- 68 g

## Cheery Charlie Checker

Servings: 2
Cooking Time: 5 Minutes
**Ingredients:**
- 1 cup skim milk
- 1 cup frozen blueberries
- 1 fresh banana
- ¾ cup plain low-fat Greek yogurt
- ½ cup frozen cherries
- ½ cup frozen strawberries
- 1 tablespoon chia seeds

**Directions:**
1. Add all the ingredients except vegetables/fruits first
2. Blend until smooth
3. Add the vegetable/fruits
4. Blend until smooth
5. Add a few ice cubes and serve the smoothie
6. Enjoy!

**Nutrition Info:** Calories: 162; Fat: 1g; Carbohydrates: 33g; Protein: 8g

# BEAUTY SMOOTHIES

## Saffron Oats Smoothie

Servings: 2-3
Cooking Time: 5 Minutes
**Ingredients:**
- 2 ripe banana, sliced (fresh or frozen)
- 1 cup fresh coconut water
- 1 teaspoon raw organic honey
- 2 tablespoons oats
- ½ teaspoon vanilla extract
- A pinch of saffron
- ½ teaspoon of almond or cashew flakes (optional)

**Directions:**
1. Place everything in the blender jar, secure the lid and pulse until smooth.

**Nutrition Info:** (Per Serving): Calories- 136, Fat- 1.2 g, Protein- 1.3 g, Carbohydrates- 33 g

## Chocolate Shake Smoothie

Servings: 2
Cooking Time: 5 Minutes
**Ingredients:**
- 1 ½ cups unsweetened almond milk
- 6 teaspoons raw organic cacao powder
- 4 tablespoons Chia seeds, soaked
- 1 teaspoon vanilla extract
- 5 teaspoons raw, organic honey
- A small pinch of cinnamon powder
- 3-4 ice cubes

**Directions:**
1. Combine all the ingredients in your high speed blender and puree until it is thick and creamy.

**Nutrition Info:** (Per Serving): Calories- 428, Fat- 15 g, Protein- 10 g, Carbohydrates- 70 g

## Bluberry Cucumber Cooler

Servings: 2
Cooking Time: 5 Minutes
**Ingredients:**
- 1 cup whole blueberries (fresh or frozen)
- 1 cup unsweetened almond milk
- ½ cup cucumber, chopped
- 2 large lettuce leaves
- 2 teaspoons hemp seeds
- 1 teaspoon raw organic honey (optional)
- 3-4 ice cubes

**Directions:**
1. Place all the ingredients into your blender and whirr it on high for 20 seconds or until the desired consistency has been reached. Pour into glasses and serve immediately.

**Nutrition Info:** (Per Serving): Calories- 202, Fat- 7.2 g, Protein- 6 g, Carbohydrates- 30 g

## Nutty Raspberry Avocado Blend

Servings: 2
Cooking Time: 5 Minutes

**Ingredients:**
- 1 cup whole raspberries (fresh or frozen)
- 3/4 cup avocado, peeled, pitted and chopped
- 3/4 cup cashews, soaked
- 1 tablespoon organic coconut oil
- 1 ½ - 2 cups filtered water
- A pinch of Himalayan salt

**Directions:**
1.  Dump all the ingredients into the blender and whip it up until the smoothie is thick and creamy.

**Nutrition Info:** (Per Serving): Calories- 698, Fat- 54 g, Protein- 9.1 g, Carbohydrates- 53 g

## Ultimate Super Food Smoothie

Servings: 3
Cooking Time: 5 Minutes
**Ingredients:**
- 1 cup unsweetened almond milk
- ¼ cup plain Greek yogurt
- ½ cup blueberries (fresh or frozen)
- ½ cup strawberries (fresh or frozen)
- 1 small ripe banana (fresh or frozen)
- A teaspoon coconut oil
- 1 ½ teaspoon bee pollen
- 1 teaspoon flax seeds
- 1 teaspoon Chia seed (soaked )
- 1 teaspoon fresh, pure Aloe Vera gel
- 1 teaspoon any other super food like maca, cacao, Hemp, Spirulina, wheatgrass, camu etc
- A few drops of liquid Stevia or agave nectar (optional)
- A pinch of cinnamon
- 4-5 ice cubes (optional)

**Directions:**
1.  Whizz up all the ingredients in the high speed blender until smooth and serve immediately.

**Nutrition Info:** (Per Serving): Calories- 345, Fat- 17.6 g, Protein- 6.2 g, Carbohydrates- 45 g

## Kale And Pomegranate Smoothie

Servings: 3
Cooking Time: 5 Minutes
**Ingredients:**
- 2/3 cup freshly prepared pomegranate juice
- 1/3 cup unsweetened almond milk
- 1 cup fresh kale, stems removed and chopped
- ¼ cup blueberries (fresh or frozen)
- ¼ cup raspberries (fresh or frozen)
- 1 ripe banana, chopped
- A handful of mixed greens
- 1 tablespoon of hemp seeds
- 1 teaspoon agave nectar
- 1 cup filtered water
- 3-4 ice cubes

**Directions:**
1.  Place all the above ingredients into the blender jar and process until the mixture is thick and creamy.

**Nutrition Info:** (Per Serving): Calories- 185, Fat- 0.5 g, Protein- 3.5 g, Carbohydrates- 40 g

# Aloe Berry Smoothie

Servings: 2
Cooking Time: 2 Minutes
**Ingredients:**
- ½ cup blueberries (fresh or frozen)
- 1/3 cup fresh and pure aloe gel or aloe Vera juice
- 2 tablespoons avocado flesh
- A handful of dandelion greens, chopped
- 1 kiwi, peeled and chopped
- 1 teaspoon coconut oil
- 1 teaspoon cacao powder
- A pinch of Celtic salt
- 1 ½ teaspoons of raw organic honey
- 1 cup filtered water

**Directions:**
1. Combine all the ingredients in a blender, secure the lid firmly and blitz until smooth.

**Nutrition Info:** (Per Serving): Calories- 305, Fat- 15 g, Protein- 2.1 g, Carbohydrates- 45 g

# All In 1 Smoothie

Servings: 2-3
Cooking Time: 5 Minutes
**Ingredients:**
- ½ cup freshly squeezed orange juice
- 1 cup carrots, peeled and chopped
- 1 cup fresh mixed greens of your choice
- 1 cup mixed berries (fresh or frozen)
- 1 small banana, copped (fresh or frozen)
- ½ cup plain low fat yogurt
- 2-3 drops of vanilla extract
- 1 teaspoon freshly squeezed lemon juice
- 3-4 ice cubes

**Directions:**
1. Pour all the ingredients into your blender and process until smooth.

**Nutrition Info:** (Per Serving): Calories- 160, Fat- 1.2 g, Protein- 5.3 g, Carbohydrates- 35 g

# Pink Potion

Servings: 3-4
Cooking Time: 5 Minutes
**Ingredients:**
- 2 cups raw beet, peeled and chopped
- 2 cups whole strawberries (fresh or frozen)
- 2 tablespoons almond butter
- 2 fresh kale leaves stems removed and chopped
- 1 banana, sliced (fresh or frozen)
- 1 teaspoon vanilla extract
- 1 tablespoon hemp seeds
- 1 cup filtered water

**Directions:**
1. Place all the ingredients into the blender and whiz up until the smoothie is nice and thick.

**Nutrition Info:** (Per Serving): Calories- 285, Fat- 11 g, Protein- 9.9 g, Carbohydrates- 40 g

# Pink Grapefruit Skin

Servings: 3
Cooking Time: 5 Minutes
**Ingredients:**
- 1 cups pineapple, chopped
- 1 small grapefruit, peeled and chopped
- 1 cups cucumber, chopped
- A handful of cilantro, washed and chopped
- ¾ cups freshly squeezed orange juice
- Freshly squeezed juice of ½ lime
- ½ teaspoon vanilla extract
- A pinch of cinnamon powder
- A pinch of sea salt
- ½ teaspoon raw organic honey
- 3-4 ice cubes

**Directions:**
1. Place all the above ingredients into the blender jar and process until the mixture is thick and creamy.

**Nutrition Info:** (Per Serving): Calories- 44, Fat- 0.5 g, Protein- 1 g, Carbohydrates- 9.1g

# Berry Dessert Smoothie

Servings: 2
Cooking Time: 5 Minutes
**Ingredients:**
- ¼ cup unsweetened almond milk
- 1 cup low fat plain yogurt
- 1 cup strawberries (fresh or frozen)
- 1 cup blueberries (fresh or frozen)
- 1 large banana, chopped(fresh or frozen)
- 1 teaspoon freshly squeezed lemon juice
- ¼ teaspoon cinnamon powder
- 3-4 ice cubes

**Directions:**
1. Place all the above ingredients into the blender jar and process until the mixture is thick and creamy.

**Nutrition Info:** (Per Serving): Calories- 265, Fat- 3.8 g, Protein- 10 g, Carbohydrates- 50 g

# Grape And Strawberry Smoothie

Servings: 2
Cooking Time: 5 Minutes
**Ingredients:**
- ½ cup whole strawberries (fresh or frozen)
- ½ cup red grapes, seedless
- 1 cup baby spinach, washed
- 1 cup mixed greens
- 2 tablespoons avocado flesh
- 2 teaspoons almond butter
- 1 teaspoon flax seed powder
- ¼ cup freshly squeezed lemon juice
- ¾ cup filtered water
- 2-3 ice cubes

**Directions:**
1. Whizz all the ingredients in the blender until smooth and serve.

**Nutrition Info:** (Per Serving): Calories- 310, Fat- 2 g, Protein- 8 g, Carbohydrates- 26 g

## Berry Beautiful Glowing Skin Smoothie

Servings: 2
Cooking Time: 5 Minutes
**Ingredients:**
- 1 cup blueberries (fresh or frozen)
- ½ cup raspberries (fresh or frozen)
- ½ cup strawberries (fresh or frozen)
- A handful of fresh kale, stems removed and chopped
- ¾ cup of plain Greek yogurt
- 2 teaspoon of raw organic honey
- 2 teaspoons freshly squeezed lemon juice
- 3 teaspoons flaxseed powder
- 4-5 ice cubes

**Directions:**
1. Pour all the ingredients into your blender and process until smooth.

**Nutrition Info:** (Per Serving): Calories- 161, Fat- 1.3 g, Protein- 8.9 g, Carbohydrates- 32 g


## Orange- Green Tonic

Servings: 1 Large
Cooking Time: 2 Minutes
**Ingredients:**
- ¾ cup mango, chopped
- ½ cup freshly squeezed orange juice
- ¾ cup fresh kale, stems removed and chopped
- 1-2 celery stalks, chopped
- 2 tablespoons fresh parsley
- 5-6 fresh mint
- 4-5 ice cubes

**Directions:**
1. Just add all the ingredients into the blender, secure the lid and whizz it up until nice and smooth.

**Nutrition Info:** (Per Serving): Calories- 160, Fat- 0.7 g, Protein- 4.3 g, Carbohydrates- 38.5 g


## Crunchy Kale – Chia Smoothie

Servings: 3-4
Cooking Time: 5 Minutes
**Ingredients:**
- 1 cup fresh kale, stems removed and chopped
- A large handful of strawberries (fresh or frozen)
- A large handful of raspberries (fresh or frozen)
- ¼ cup red bell pepper, deseeded and chopped
- 1 ½ cups unsweetened almond milk
- 1 cup fresh coconut water
- 1 ½ teaspoon Chia seeds
- 6-7 whole almonds , soaked

**Directions:**
1. Add all the above ingredients into your blender jar and pulse until thick and frothy.

**Nutrition Info:** (Per Serving): Calories- 234, Fat- 21.5 g, Protein- 3 g, Carbohydrates- 21 g

# Min-tea Mango Rejuvinating Smoothie

Servings: 2
Cooking Time: 5 Minutes

**Ingredients:**

- ½ cup freshly brewed green tea (1/2 cup water+ 1 tea bag)
- ½ cup baby spinach, washed and chopped
- ½ cup mangos, cooped
- 1 teaspoon pure coconut oil
- 4-5 fresh mint leaves
- A tiny pinch of sea salt
- 1 teaspoon of freshly squeezed lemon juice

**Directions:**

1. Add all the above ingredients into your blender jar and pulse until thick and frothy.

**Nutrition Info:** (Per Serving): Calories- 234, Fat- 21 g, Protein- 3.3 g, Carbohydrates-32 g

# ENERGY BOOSTING SMOOTHIES

## Green Skinny Energizer

Servings: 2
Cooking Time: 5 Minutes
**Ingredients:**
- ½ ripe mango, pitted and sliced
- 1 cup kale, chopped
- 3 cups baby spinach
- 1 cup coconut water

**Directions:**
1. Add all the ingredients except vegetables/fruits first
2. Blend until smooth
3. Add the vegetable/fruits
4. Blend until smooth
5. Add a few ice cubes and serve the smoothie
6. Enjoy!

**Nutrition Info:** Calories: 300; Fat: 13g; Carbohydrates: 37g; Protein: 10g

## Dandelion And Carrot Booster

Servings: 2
Cooking Time: 5 Minutes
**Ingredients:**
- ½ fuji apple
- 1 tablespoon fresh ginger
- ½ pound organic carrots, scrubbed
- ¾ cup dandelion greens
- 2 cups baby spinach

**Directions:**
1. Add all the ingredients except vegetables/fruits first
2. Blend until smooth
3. Add the vegetable/fruits
4. Blend until smooth
5. Add a few ice cubes and serve the smoothie
6. Enjoy!

**Nutrition Info:** Calories: 160; Fat: 5g; Carbohydrates: 30g; Protein: 5g

## Apple- Date Smoothie

Servings: 3
Cooking Time: 5 Minutes
**Ingredients:**
- 2 large apples, peeled , cored and chopped
- 1 large ripe banana, chopped
- 3 tablespoons almond butter or cashew butter
- 4-5 collard greens, stems removed and chopped
- 2-3 medjool dates, pitted
- 3 teaspoons hemp powder
- 1 ½ cups filtered water

**Directions:**
1. Place all the ingredients into your high speed blender jar and pulse it for 30 seconds until everything is well combined.

**Nutrition Info:** (Per Serving): Calories- 481, Fat- 20 g, Protein- 12.2 g, Carbohydrates- 73.5 g

# Mango Beet Energy Booster

Servings: 2
Cooking Time: 5 Minutes
**Ingredients:**
- ½ cup unsweetened almond milk
- 1 cup red beet, peeled and chopped
- 1 ripe banana, chopped (fresh or frozen)
- 1 small mango, peeled and chopped
- 2 cups baby spinach, chopped
- ½ teaspoon freshly grated giber
- A handful of ice cubes

**Directions:**
1. Load your blender with all the ingredients mentioned above and run it on medium high for 45 seconds until there are no lumps. Pour into beautiful glasses and serve.

**Nutrition Info:** (Per Serving): Calories- 165, Fat- 1.1 g, Protein- 4 g, Carbohydrates- 40 g

# Matcha And Lettuce Booster

Servings: 3
Cooking Time: 5 Minutes
**Ingredients:**
- 2 cups unsweetened almond milk
- 1 cup fresh romaine lettuce, washed and chopped
- 2 ripe bananas (fresh or frozen)
- 1 tablespoon Matcha powder
- 1 teaspoon raw organic honey
- 1 teaspoon freshly squeezed lemon juice
- 3-4 ice cubes

**Directions:**
1. To your blender jar, add all the items and un it for 45 seconds on medium high speed. Pit into serving glasses and enjoy.

**Nutrition Info:** (Per Serving): Calories- 250, Fat- 10 g, Protein- 6.2 g, Carbohydrates- 36 g

# Ginger- Pomegranate Smoothie

Servings: 2
Cooking Time: 2 Minutes
**Ingredients:**
- 1 cup freshly prepared homemade pomegranate juice
- 4 ounces of plain Greek yogurt
- 1 large banana, chopped (fresh or frozen)
- ¼ teaspoon freshly grated ginger
- 1 teaspoon freshly squeezed lemon juice
- 3-4 ice cubes

**Directions:**
1. Pour all the ingredients into the blender and puree until smooth and frothy.

**Nutrition Info:** (Per Serving): Calories- 192, Fat- 2.1 g, Protein- 7.8 g, Carbohydrates- 40 g

# Orange Antioxidant Refresher

Servings: 2
Cooking Time: 5 Minutes
**Ingredients:**
- 4 ounces pineapple

- 1 orange, peeled
- 1 teaspoon pomegranate powder
- 1 mini orange, peeled
- ½ teaspoon turmeric
- ½ teaspoon ginger
- 1 cup ice
- 1 cup of water

**Directions:**
1. Add all the listed ingredients to a blender
2. Blend until you have a smooth and creamy texture
3. Serve chilled and enjoy!

**Nutrition Info:** Calories: 101; Fat: 1g; Carbohydrates: 25g; Protein: 2g

## Apple Mulberry Smoothie

Servings: 2
Cooking Time: 5 Minutes
**Ingredients:**
- 1 cup mulberries (fresh or frozen)
- 1 large banana, chipped 9fresh or frozen)
- 1 cup fresh, homemade apple juice (or 2 apples, cored and chopped)
- 1 cup fresh kale, stems removed
- 5 tablespoons rolled oats
- 3 tablespoons chopped cashews
- 1 teaspoon vanilla extract

**Directions:**
1. Add everything to your blender jar, secure the lid and whizz it on high for 30 seconds until the desired consistency is reached, pour into glasses and serve.

**Nutrition Info:** (Per Serving): Calories- 387, Fat- 18 g, Protein- 31 g, Carbohydrates- 30 g

## Coconut- Flaxseed Smoothie

Servings: 1
Cooking Time: 2 Minutes
**Ingredients:**
- 1 cup fresh coconut water
- 1 small bananas, chopped
- 4 spinach leaves, washed and chopped
- ½ cup whole strawberries (fresh or frozen)
- 1 tablespoon flaxseed powder
- 3-4 ice cubes

**Directions:**
1. Load all the ingredients into the blender and whiz until smooth.

**Nutrition Info:** (Per Serving): Calories- 300, Fat- 4.2 g, Protein- 6.2 g, Carbohydrates- 67 g

## Coco-nana Smoothie

Servings: 1 Large
Cooking Time: 2 Minutes
**Ingredients:**
- ¾ cup fresh coconut water
- A handful of whole strawberries (fresh or frozen)
- 1 ripe banana (fresh or frozen)
- A handful of spinach leaves
- 1 teaspoon of flax seed powder
- 2-3 ice cubes (optional)

**Directions:**

1. Pour all the ingredients in the blender and pulse until there are no lumps. Pour into glasses and enjoy.
**Nutrition Info:** (Per Serving): Calories- 145, Fat- 2.2 g, Protein- 3.1 g, Carbohydrates- 32 g

## Powerful Green Frenzy

Servings: 2
Cooking Time: 5 Minutes
**Ingredients:**
- 1 cup ice
- 2 tablespoons almond butter
- 1 teaspoon spirulina
- 3 teaspoons fresh ginger
- 1½ frozen bananas, sliced
- 2 cups baby spinach, chopped
- 1 cup kale
- 1½ cups unsweetened almond milk

**Directions:**
1. Add all the ingredients except vegetables/fruits first
2. Blend until smooth
3. Add the vegetable/fruits
4. Blend until smooth
5. Add a few ice cubes and serve the smoothie
6. Enjoy!

**Nutrition Info:** Calories: 350; Fat: 4g; Carbohydrates: 54g; Protein: 30g

## Grape And Green Tea Smoothie

Servings: 2-3
Cooking Time: 20 Minutes
**Ingredients:**
- 1 ½ cups freshly brewed green tea
- A handful of baby spinach, washed and chopped
- 1 cup kale, stems removed and chopped
- ½ cup green grapes( seedless)
- ½ avocado, peeled and chopped
- 1 ripe banana, chopped (fresh or frozen)
- 2 teaspoons Chia seeds, soaked for 15 minutes
- 2-3 ice cubes

**Directions:**
1. Place all the items into the blender jar, secure the lid firmly and process until the smoothie has reached the desired consistency.

**Nutrition Info:** (Per Serving): Calories- 160, Fat- 6.7, Protein- 3.8 g, Carbohydrates- 20 g

## Energizing Pineapple Kicker

Servings: 2
Cooking Time: 5 Minutes
**Ingredients:**
- 1 medium cucumber, diced
- ¾ cup fresh pineapple
- 1 tablespoon fresh ginger
- 3 cups baby spinach

**Directions:**
1. Add all the ingredients except vegetables/fruits first
2. Blend until smooth
3. Add the vegetable/fruits
4. Blend until smooth
5. Add a few ice cubes and serve the smoothie

6.    Enjoy!
**Nutrition Info:** Calories: 236; Fat: 6g; Carbohydrates: 46g; Protein: 4g

## Berry- Mint Cooler

Servings: 2
Cooking Time: 2 Minutes
**Ingredients:**
- 2 cups unsweetened almond milk
- A large handful of frozen blueberries
- 1 ½ teaspoons of raw, organic honey
- 1 ½ teaspoon flax seed powder
- 3-4 fresh mint leaves
- 4-5 ice cubes

**Directions:**
1.    To your high speed blender, add all the ingredients and process for 30 seconds or until done.
**Nutrition Info:** (Per Serving): Calories- 201, Fat-7.2 g, Protein-11 g, Carbohydrates- 21 g

## Verry- Berry Breakfast

Servings: 2
Cooking Time: 2 Minutes
**Ingredients:**
- ¾ cup unsweetened almond milk
- ½ large banana, chopped
- ¾ cup plain Greek yogurt
- 1 cup mixed berries (fresh or frozen)
- ½ teaspoon raw organic honey (optional)
- 3-5 ice cubes

**Directions:**
1.    Place all the above ingredients into your high speed blender and process for 45 seconds on medium high speed till the smoothie is thick and creamy.
**Nutrition Info:** (Per Serving): Calories- 255, Fat- 1.2 g, Protein- 26 g, Carbohydrates- 42 g

## Pumpkin Seed And Yogurt Smoothie

Servings: 2
Cooking Time: 5 Minutes
**Ingredients:**
- 1 cup plain Greek yogurt
- 1 cup freshly squeezed grapefruit juice
- 1 avocado, peeled, pitted and chopped
- 2 cups fresh kale, stems removed
- 3 teaspoons almond butter
- 3 teaspoons pumpkin seeds
- ½ cup filtered water

**Directions:**
1.    Add all the ingredients into the blender jar and whirr it up until nice and smooth.
**Nutrition Info:** (Per Serving): Calories- 432, Fat- 32 g, Protein- 17g, Carbohydrates- 42 g

# DIABETES SMOOTHIES

## Simple Strawberry Smoothie

Servings: 1
Cooking Time: 2 Minutes
**Ingredients:**
- 1 cup unsweetened almond milk
- 6 whole strawberries (fresh or frozen)
- 4 ounces plain Greek yogurt
- ¼ teaspoon vanilla extract
- 4-5 ice cubes

**Directions:**
1. Add the liquids, ice, vanilla and berries into the blender and process it on medium speed for 30 seconds or until thick and creamy.

**Nutrition Info:** (Per Serving): Calories- 165, Fat- 6 g, Protein- 15 g, Carbohydrates- 12 g

## Spicy Pear And Green Tea

Servings: 2
Cooking Time: 5 Minutes
**Ingredients:**
- 1 cup brewed and chilled green tea
- ½ cup silken tofu
- 1 small pear, skin on, cut into small pieces
- ½ frozen bananas, sliced into rounds
- 2 tablespoons ground flaxseed
- 1/8 teaspoon cayenne
- 2 tablespoons lemon juice
- ½ cup ice

**Directions:**
1. Add all the ingredients except vegetables/fruits first
2. Blend until smooth
3. Add the vegetable/fruits
4. Blend until smooth
5. Add a few ice cubes and serve the smoothie
6. Enjoy!

**Nutrition Info:** Calories: 422; Fat: 13g; Carbohydrates: 51g; Protein: 31g

## Pineapple Broccoli Smoothie

Servings: 2
Cooking Time: 10 Minutes
**Ingredients:**
- 1 cup strawberries
- 2 cups almond milk
- 2 cups broccoli florets
- ½ cup pineapple
- 2 teaspoons honey

**Directions:**
1. Add listed ingredients to a blender
2. Blend until you have a smooth and creamy texture
3. Serve chilled and enjoy!

**Nutrition Info:** Calories: 324; Fat: 25.4g; Carbohydrates: 18g; Protein: 4.3g

## Diabetic Berry Blast

Servings: 1
Cooking Time: 10 Minutes
**Ingredients:**
- 2 tablespoons flax meal
- 3 kale leaves
- 2 cups unsweetened mango chunks
- 1 cup frozen raspberries
- 1 cup frozen blackberries
- 1 cup frozen blueberries

**Directions:**
1. Add all the listed ingredients to a blender
2. Blend until you have a smooth and creamy texture
3. Serve chilled and enjoy!

**Nutrition Info:** Calories: 153; Fat: 11g; Carbohydrates: 8g; Protein: 7g

## Cherry-berry Smoothie

Servings: 2
Cooking Time: 2 Minutes
**Ingredients:**
- ¾ cup sweet or sour cherries (fresh or frozen)
- ¼ cup blueberries (fresh or frozen)
- ½ cup unsweetened almond milk
- 1 cup plain Greek yogurt
- 1 large banana, chopped (fresh or frozen)
- ½ teaspoon vanilla extract
- 3-4 ice cubes

**Directions:**
1. Add everything to your blender and pulse it on high for 20 seconds and your smoothie is ready. Enjoy!

**Nutrition Info:** (Per Serving): Calories- 105, Fat- 1.2 g, Protein- 5.1 g, Carbohydrates-22 g

## Hemp And Kale Smoothie

Servings: 2
Cooking Time: 5 Minutes
**Ingredients:**
- 1 large banana, chopped (fresh or frozen)
- A large handful of baby spinach, washed and chopped
- A large handful of kale, stems removed and chopped
- 1 tablespoon of hemp seeds
- 2-3 drops of liquid Stevia (optional)
- 2 teaspoons of freshly squeezed lemon juice
- 1 ½ cups of filtered water

**Directions:**
1. Place all the ingredients in the blender jar, secure the lid and pulse it for 20 seconds until everything is well combined.

**Nutrition Info:** (Per Serving): Calories- 340, Fat- 16 g, Protein- 15 g, Carbohydrates- 44 g

## Lime "n" Lemony Cucumber Cooler

Servings: 3
Cooking Time: 5 Minutes
**Ingredients:**

- 2 cups plain fat free yogurt
- 2 cups green cucumber, chopped
- 1 green pear, cored and chopped
- Freshly squeezed juice of 1 lime
- 1 tablespoon freshly squeezed lemon juice
- 2-3 ice cubes

**Directions:**
1. Place all the ingredients into the high speed blender and blitz until thick and creamy. Serve immediately!

**Nutrition Info:** (Per Serving): Calories- 175, Fat- 4.2 g, Protein- 11 g, Carbohydrates- 63 g

## Coconut -mint Smoothie

Servings: 2
Cooking Time: 5 Minutes
**Ingredients:**
- 1 cup mango, chopped
- 1 cup fresh kale, stems removed and chopped
- A handful of lettuce
- 1-2 celery stalks
- ½ cup fresh mint, washed and chopped
- ½ cup Italian flat leafed parsley, washed
- 2 teaspoon coconut oil
- ¾ cup coconut water

**Directions:**
1. Place everything into the blender, secure the lid and process until smooth.

**Nutrition Info:** (Per Serving): Calories-220, Fat- 15 g, 4.1 g, Protein- Carbohydrates- 25 g

## The Great Dia Green Smoothie

Servings: 1
Cooking Time: 10 Minutes
**Ingredients:**
- 1 whole banana
- 1 cup kale
- 1 cup spinach
- 2 tablespoons chia seeds, soaked
- A handful of mixed berries

**Directions:**
1. Add all the listed ingredients to a blender
2. Blend until you have a smooth and creamy texture
3. Serve chilled and enjoy!

**Nutrition Info:** Calories: 180; Fat: 15g; Carbohydrates: 8g; Protein: 5g

## Cacao – Avocado Smoothie

Servings: 1 Large
Cooking Time: 2 Minutes
**Ingredients:**
- 1 cup organic coconut milk
- 4 teaspoons cacao powder
- ½ avocado, peeled, pitted and chopped
- 4-5 drops liquid Stevia (optional)
- 1 teaspoon Chia seeds
- 4-5 ice cubes

**Directions:**
1. Add everything into the blender jar and process until nice and thick.
**Nutrition Info:** (Per Serving): Calories- 285, Fat- 23 g, Protein- 8 g, Carbohydrates- 23 g

## Healthy Potato Pie Glass

Servings: 2
Cooking Time: 5 Minutes
**Ingredients:**
- 1 cup ice
- ¼ teaspoon cinnamon
- ¼ cup rolled oats
- ½ frozen banana
- 1 small orange, peeled
- ½ cup sweet potato, cooked and peeled
- 6 ounces Greek yogurt
- ½ cup unsweetened almond milk

**Directions:**
1. Add all the ingredients except vegetables/fruits first
2. Blend until smooth
3. Add the vegetable/fruits
4. Blend until smooth
5. Add a few ice cubes and serve the smoothie
6. Enjoy!
**Nutrition Info:** Calories: 400; Fat: 20g; Carbohydrates: 41g; Protein: 20g

## White Bean And Mango Delight

Servings: 2
Cooking Time: 5 Minutes
**Ingredients:**
- 1 cup ice
- 2 tablespoons fresh mint leaves, chopped
- 1 tablespoon coconut flour
- 2 tablespoons hemp seeds
- ½ cup frozen spinach
- ½ cup frozen mango
- 1/3 cup white beans, rinsed
- 1 cup cashew milk

**Directions:**
1. Add all the ingredients except vegetables/fruits first
2. Blend until smooth
3. Add the vegetable/fruits
4. Blend until smooth
5. Add a few ice cubes and serve the smoothie
6. Enjoy!
**Nutrition Info:** Calories: 290; Fat: 10g; Carbohydrates: 37g; Protein: 12g

# Appendix : Recipes Index

Peachyfig Green Smoothie 40
Peanut Butter Berry Smoothie 25
Peanut Butter Broccoli Smoothie 28
Pear-simmon Smoothie 38
Pina Berry Smoothie 32
Pina Colada Smoothie 84
Pineapple & Almond Smoothie 60
Pineapple & Coconut Smoothie 59
Pineapple And Cucumber Cooler 79
Pineapple Broccoli Smoothie 104
Pineapple Papaya Perfection Smoothie 27
Pineapple Protein Smoothie 18
Pineapple Sage Smoothie 64
Pink Grapefruit Skin 96
Pink Potion 95
Pomegranate- Berry Smoothie 8
Popoye's Pear Smoothie For Kids 7
Powerful Green Frenzy 102
Powerful Kale And Carrot Glass 48
Protein-packed Root Beer Shake 19
Punkin Seed And Yogurt Smoothie 103

**R**

Raspberry And White Chocolate Shake 20
Raspberry Carrot Smoothie 71
Raspberry Flaxseed Smoothie 55
Raspberry- Grapefruit Smoothie 22
Raspberry Peach Delight 70
Raspberry Pecan Date Delight 30
Raspberry Smoothie 82
Rasp-ricot Smoothie 40
Raw Chocolate Smoothie 30
Red Healing Potion 38

**S**

Saffron Oats Smoothie 93
Sapodilla, Chia And Almond Milk Smoothie 56
Simple Anti-aging Cacao Dream 49
Simple Cherry Berry Wonder 46
Simple Strawberry Smoothie 104
Snicker Doodle Smoothie 18
Spiced Banana Smoothie 63
Spiced Blackberry Smoothie 50
Spiced Peach Smoothie 61
Spiced Pineapple Smoothie 22
Spicy Pear And Green Tea 104
Spinach & Berries Smoothie 59
Spinach And Grape Smoothie 33
Spinach And Kiwi Smoothie 66
Spinach, Grape, & Coconut Smoothie 82
Spin-apple Pear Smoothie 54

Straight Up Avocado And Kale Smoothie 24
Strawberry And Watermelon Medley 11
Strawberry Coconut Snowflake 20
Strawberry Watermelon Smoothie 85
Strawberry-ginger Tea Smoothie 5
Sunrise Smoothie 22
Super Avocado Smoothie 83
Super Duper Berry Smoothie 49
Super Tropi-kale Wonder 72
Super Veggie Smoothie 46
Sweet And Spicy Fruit Punch 61
Sweet Pea Smoothie 91
Sweet Protein And Cherry Shake 19

**T**

Tangy Ginger & Radish Smoothie 59
Tea And Grape Smoothie 74
The Anti-aging Avocado 47
The Anti-aging Superfood Glass 47
The Blueberry And Chocolate Delight 29
The Cacao Super Smoothie 18
The Great Avocado And Almond Delight 16
The Great Dia Green Smoothie 106
The Nutty Macadamia Delight 57
The Pinky Swear 43
The Pumpkin Eye 55
The Wisest Watermelon Glass 90
Tomato- Melon Refreshing Smoothie 53
Tropical Matcha Kale 75
Turmeric-mango Smoothie 62
Twisty Cucumber Honeydew 12

**U**

Ultimate Berry Blush 31
Ultimate Cold And Flu Fighting Smoothie 5
Ultimate Orange Potion 51
Ultimate Super Food Smoothie 94

**V**

Vanilla- Mango Madness 32
Vanilla-oats Smoothie 55
Verry- Berry Breakfast 103
Verry-berry Carrot Delight 32
Very Berry Blueberry Wonder 30
Very-berry Orange 15

**W**

White Bean And Mango Delight 107

**Y**

Yogi- Banana Agave Smoothie 41
Yogi-berry Smoothie 8
Zucchini Apple Smoothie 24

CPSIA information can be obtained
at www.ICGtesting.com
Printed in the USA
BVHW010216280521
608367BV00012B/286